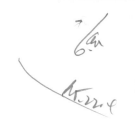

THE HEART
AND CIRCULATORY SYSTEM

YOUR BODY YOUR HEALTH

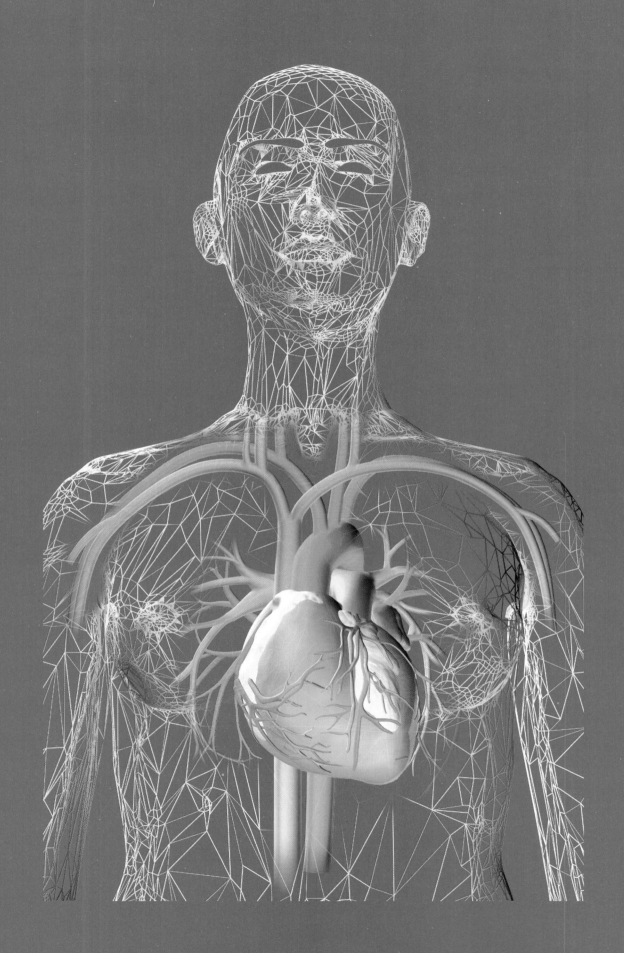

THE HEART
AND CIRCULATORY SYSTEM

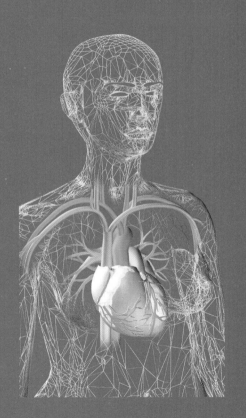
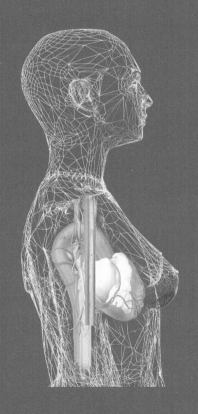
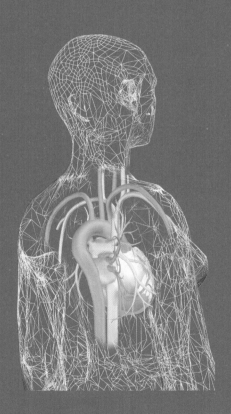

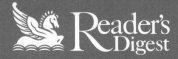
Reader's
Digest

The Reader's Digest Association, Inc.
Pleasantville, New York
London Sydney Montreal

The Heart and Circulatory System

was created and produced by
Carroll & Brown Limited
20 Lonsdale Road
London NW6 6RD

Library of Congress Cataloging-in-Publication
Data has been applied for.

ISBN 0-7621-0437-6

Printed in the United States of America
1 3 5 7 9 8 6 4 2

The information in this book is for
reference only; it is not intended as a
substitute for a doctor's diagnosis and
care. The editors urge anyone with
continuing medical problems or
symptoms to consult a doctor.

American Edition Produced by

NOVA Graphic Services, Inc.
501 Office Center Drive, Suite 190
Ft. Washington, PA 19034 USA
(215)542-3900

President
David Davenport

Editorial Director
Robin C. Bonner

Composition Manager
Steve Magnin

Art Director
Karen Kappe

Cardiology Specialist Consultant
Dr. Nirav N. Mehta, MD, Cardiologist,
Thomas Jefferson University, Philadelphia

CONTRIBUTORS

Dr Adrian P Banning

Dr Aidan Buckley, MRCP, Department of Cardiology, Aberdeen Royal Infirmary, Aberdeen

Mr Michele de Bonis, MD, Department of Cardiac Surgery,
San Raffaele University Hospital, Milan

Mr Josh Derodra, MB BS, FRCS, MS, Department of Vascular Surgery, Medway Hospital

Dr Duncan Hogg, MB, ChB, MRCP,
British Heart Foundation, Department of Cardiology, Aberdeen Royal Infirmary, Aberdeen

Fiona Hunter, BSc, Dip, Dietitian

Dr Andrew D Kelion, MA, MRCP, Cardiology Department, John Radcliffe Hospital, Oxford

Joel Levy, BSc, MA, Freelance Medical Writer

Dr Chris Plummer, BSc, PhD, BM, BCh, MRCP, Department of Cardiology,
Freeman Hospital, Newcastle Upon Tyne

Helen Stracey, BSc, SRD, State Registered Dietitian

Karan Thomas, BSc, Physical Activity and Health Specialist

Dr Hamish Walker, MRCP, Department of Cardiology, Hammersmith Hospital, London

Dr Hazel White, BA, MB, BChir, Yorkshire Heart Centre, Leeds

Dr Zaheer Yousef, BSc, MB BS, MCRP
Department of Cardiology, The Rayne Institute, St. Thomas' Hospital, London

For the Reader's Digest
Editor in Chief Neil E. Wertheimer
Editorial Director Christopher Cavanaugh
Senior Designer Judith Carmel
Production Technology Manager Douglas A. Croll
Manufacturing Manager John L. Cassidy

The Heart and Circulatory System

Awareness of health issues and expectations of medicine are greater today than ever before. A long and healthy life has come to be looked on not so much as a matter of luck but almost as a right. However, as our knowledge of health and the causes of disease has grown, it has become increasingly clear that health is something that we can all influence, for better or worse, through choices we make in our lives. *Your Body Your Health* is designed to help you make the right choices to make the most of your health potential. Each volume in the series focuses on a different physiological system of the body, explaining what it does and how it works. In each, you will find a wealth of advice and health tips on diet, exercise, and lifestyle factors, as well as the health checks you can expect throughout life. You will find out what can go wrong and what can be done about it, and you will learn from people's real-life experiences of diagnosis and treatment. Finally, a detailed A to Z index includes major conditions that can affect the system. The series builds into a complete user's manual for the care and maintenance of the entire body.

This volume looks at the heart—the driving force behind your body—and its associated circulatory system. No other organ is so immensely hard-working, or is forced to endure so much strain from the excesses of modern life. Here we reveal the remarkable design of your heart, from the structure of its chambers and valves to the electrical system that controls the split-second timing of its pumping action. Find out how it delivers vital oxygen and nutrients to your body, every second of every day—and learn how to protect it. Read how you can lessen your risk of heart problems by controlling certain lifestyle factors, in particular smoking and stress. Chart your way around the complexities of cholesterol, caffeine, and alcohol, and learn of the very real benefits that a regular aerobic workout can bring. You can also meet the medical experts and discover the impressive array of tools and treatments at their disposal to deal with diseases of the heart and circulatory system.

Contents

3

What happens when things go wrong

The life story of the heart

There are few sounds that are more evocative than a human heartbeat. Imprinted on your brain as the constant background noise of your months in the womb, the heartbeat symbolizes life itself. All around the world, the pulse is connected with concepts such as "life-blood" and "life-force," and there are many good reasons for these powerful associations.

Every beat of your heart drives blood through a vast network of tubes and pipes that reaches into every corner of your body, circulating blood to almost all of your 75 trillion cells (only your cornea—the transparent layer at the front of your eyes—receives no blood supply). If this circulation is interrupted for even a few minutes, the consequences can be catastrophic. Your cells, deprived of the oxygen that blood brings them, simply suffocate. Fortunately, evolution has equipped you with an amazing device for meeting your body's insatiable demand for oxygen—the human heart.

THE RHYTHM OF LIFE

The heart can justifiably claim to be the hardest working organ in the human body. Engineers and scientists marvel at its sheer endurance and can only dream of making a machine that can match its performance without disintegrating within a few years. This does not mean that the heart is especially complex nor even particularly big. Close your hand to make a fist (if you have small hands, clasp the fist in your other hand) and take a look at it—this is approximately the size of your own heart. In basic layout it is simple but ingenious: Like all the best designs, its form perfectly fits its function. Your heart is essentially a ball of muscle with four interconnecting spaces inside it. When the muscles squeeze, blood is either

A healthy heart—for life
There is nothing inevitable about heart disease if we take care of ourselves from an early age. Simple lifestyle changes will help us to live better longer.

moved between the spaces or is driven out into blood vessels that lead to the rest of the body. This may not sound too impressive, until you consider how much blood is actually pumped by the heart, day in and day out.

To fully appreciate the Herculean scale of the task undertaken by your heart, imagine using a teacup to empty a bathtub of water in just 15 minutes. Now imagine doing it nonstop, every second of every hour of every day of every year, without stopping to rest or sleep—and definitely no coffee breaks—for about 80 years. This is the task performed by the average human heart.

THE PATH TO YOUR HEART
The largest vessels start at the heart, splitting again and again until they form a web of microscopic vessels—more than 10 billion—that reaches into the farthest corners of your body. Here your blood delivers its load of oxygen and nutrients to the hungry cells and in return picks up their waste. On the return route, the tiny tubes gather together to form progressively larger vessels, leading back to the heart to complete the circulatory network.

These blood vessels form more than just a set of immobile pipes: They actively help to drive blood around your body and are amazingly responsive to the changing demands of your many tissues. For instance, the 10 billion minuscule vessels in your body, from your fingertips to your toes, can alter their width to channel blood to where it is needed most. The heart itself is capable of an amazing range of activity—During heavy exercise, for instance, it can increase its already considerable output by a factor of six and quadruple its normal rate of beating.

The heart can be seen as the body's engine, supplying the power to keep you moving and responding to signals from your body and brain—the biological equivalent of stepping on the accelerator. The circulatory system distributes power (in the form of oxygen and nutrients) to the parts of the body that need it, just as a driveshaft distributes power from the engine to the wheels. Together, the heart and circulation are known as the cardiovascular system.

A LIFE HISTORY OF YOUR HEART
How does the body develop such an efficient, powerful, and responsive system? The story begins in the womb, within days of conception. The heart is one of the first organs to appear within the developing fetus. In its first two weeks, an embryo may look like an undifferentiated blob, but it already has a defined head and tail. The heart grows from a cluster of cells just below the head end; these cells develop the ability to twitch. By the third week of pregnancy this patch has folded over into a tube, and

Your heart lies at the center of a 60,000-mile network of blood vessels. If all these vessels were laid out end to end, they would stretch almost two and a half times around the earth.

the irregular first flutterings of this "proto-heart" can be detected. After four weeks, the tube acquires kinks, which are the precursors of the division of the heart into different chambers, and the twitching of the heart cells becomes regular and synchronized. Eventually, the fetal heart will beat twice as fast as an adult's—at about 150 beats per minute (bpm). By the time the fetus is 12 weeks old, its heart is pumping on average an amazing 60 pints of blood a day.

The circulatory system forms even before the heart itself—Blood vessels first appear just 17 days after conception. As the heart tube thickens and swells during the third and fourth weeks, the major vessels leading to and from it are already present in primitive form. By the second month of gestation, all of the major blood vessels are fully formed and in place, and the fetal liver is manufacturing the blood to fill them.

By week 12 all the structures that make up the fetus are present—From now on development consists of growth and increasing specialization of tissues. The heart and circulatory system are the only parts of the body that undergo major structural changes after this point. Life in the womb requires special adaptations for the heart; there is no air to breathe, and all the necessary food and oxygen come via the umbilical cord. Shortcuts between the chambers of the heart and the major blood vessels allow the fetus to make the most efficient use of its blood. These shortcuts disappear at birth (see pages 34 to 35), and the heart begins normal operation in the pattern it will follow for roughly the next 80 years.

A newborn's heart rate, around 125 bpm, is almost twice the average adult's. Over the next 12 to 14 years, this rate gradually falls to around 70 bpm. As the body grows, the heart also increases in size, and the blood

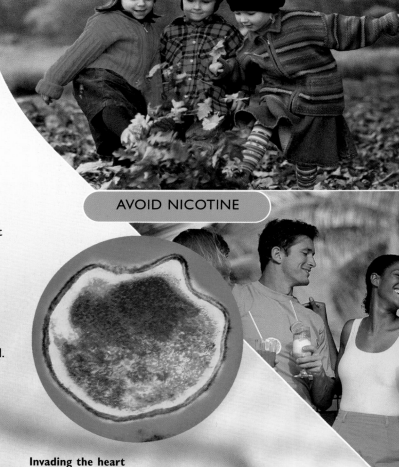

THE WAY TO A HEALTHY HEART

Research repeatedly shows that key lifestyle factors including eating a healthy, balanced diet, avoiding smoking and heavy drinking, exercising and staying active from an early age, as well as taking time to relax with your loved ones can all dramatically influence your heart health and the quality of your life.

KEEP ACTIVE

AVOID NICOTINE

Invading the heart
Smoking encourages the growth bacteria such as Chlamydia pneumoniae, *which have been linked to heart disease.*

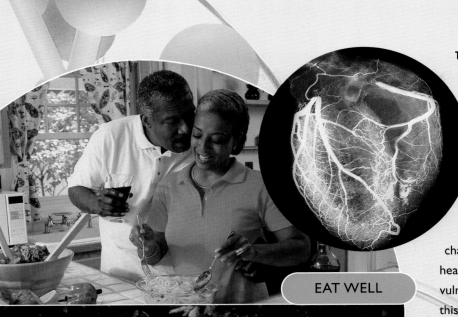

EAT WELL

The hard-working heart
Modern life puts added strain on what is already your hardest working organ.

vessels in length. By maturity, the average human heart weighs about 9½ ounces. During the next few decades it works tirelessly, but eventually age will take its toll. Subtle changes build up over time, eroding the heart's ability to function and making it vulnerable to heart attacks. The rate at which this happens, and the extent of any damage, is different for everyone.

AT THE HEART OF THE MATTER

Few aspects of health appear to be as random or capricious as the sudden, deadly heart attack. Nearly everyone knows a story of a fitness fanatic who dropped dead of a heart attack during his morning run, and many people seem to have a grandparent who has lived to a ripe old age despite smoking and drinking for many years. Why does heart health seem to be such a lottery, and what can you do about it?

Due to the combined effects of your genetic inheritance and the environmental influences that have shaped your life, your heart and circulatory system are unique. The size and strength of your heart, the elasticity of your blood vessels, their vulnerability to the build-up of deposits, and the levels of damaging substances (such as cholesterol) in your blood are all factors particular to you.

The extent to which these factors are governed by your genes is the subject of debate, but there is no doubt that heredity plays a part in determining your heart health. At present there is no way of finding out whether you are carrying genes that threaten your cardiovascular health (and there is nothing you can do to change them anyway) but this may

REDUCE STRESS

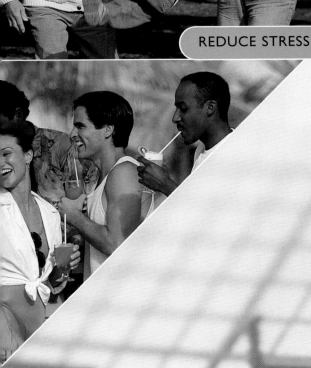

In the blood
A family history of cardiovascular problems is a warning to take extra special care of your heart: Your DNA may contain inherited genes that predispose you to heart or circulatory disease.

*The human heart pumps an amazing
1,600 gallons of blood around the body each day—
enough to fill a small swimming pool.*

change in the future. Scientists are already racing to identify heart-risk genes, and screening programs could be in place within the decade. In the meantime, there is a lot that you can do to ensure your cardiovascular health, whatever your genetic legacy. A typical Western lifestyle exposes the heart and circulatory system to numerous risks. Although your genes make you more or less vulnerable, knowing the nature of these risks will allow you to take steps to minimize them.

LISTEN TO YOUR HEART

Assessing your heart health status and developing a clear picture of your personal risk profile—the quality of your diet, your activity levels, and so on—are important first steps in developing a healthier lifestyle. Once you know where improvements can be made, you can really take charge of your heart health. Relatively straightforward lifestyle changes can have an enormous impact. For example, giving up smoking can cut your risk of cardiovascular disease in half within five years. Exercising regularly is a

Moving to a new beat
*Exercise is cheap, fun, and an
extremely effective form
of preventive medicine.*

great way to boost everything from your heart capacity to circulatory health and even mental well-being. Dramatic benefits can also be achieved through your diet. Studies show that eating a balanced diet that includes plenty of fruit and vegetables but less fat, red meat, and salt can reduce the risk of cardiovascular disease by a substantial degree. Stress, a huge problem in the developed world, can pose a range of cardiovascular health risks. Understanding the sources of your stress and learning how best to deal with them will ultimately make you a happier, as well as a healthier, person.

Cardiovascular disease is still, however, the leading cause of death in industrialized nations, and there is evidence that the vast majority of the adult population of the Western world suffer from some degree of cardiovascular ill health. For instance, autopsies on young American men who had died in car accidents revealed that virtually all of them had suffered some degree of narrowing of the arteries. In the United States, 1 in 5 adults suffers from high blood pressure (hypertension), and the figure is much higher for some ethnic groups, such as African-Americans. The numbers from some other countries are even higher. There is no doubt that cardio-vascular disease is the central health issue in the developed world.

MAINTAINING THE MACHINE
Cardiovascular diagnosis and treatment are among the most important branches of modern medicine. Drug treatments can help to control many conditions that would otherwise be life threatening, and recent advances in this field are exciting. Recent ground-breaking work has revealed the role of bacterial infection in heart disease, raising the hope that the simple antibiotic may become a force in the fight against heart disease.

When drugs fail, surgery may be necessary. Some of the most famous developments in 20th-century medicine have involved surgical procedures on the heart. Dr Christiaan Barnard captured the world's attention in 1967, when he performed the first successful heart transplant. Other milestones include implanted pacemakers, artificial blood vessels, and artificial parts for the heart. Within the next few decades, people may be able to grow a "bank" of cloned tissues to replace their own worn-out parts—blood vessels, muscle tissue, and even whole hearts.

Clearly the future holds important advances that will transform the public health landscape, but are we really prepared for their impact? For instance, screening for genes that predispose for high cholesterol levels may be available in the near future, but can we predict the consequences? If you found that your genes made you extremely tolerant of high-cholesterol foods, you might be tempted to indulge in an excess of fatty foods, damaging your health irreparably. Alternatively, the benefits of early detection could be outweighed by the stress of knowing

The nanotechnicians
Scientists hope in the future to build microscopic machines from just a few molecules; these would be capable of "sweeping" their way through a clogged-up artery to restore a free-flowing blood supply.

that you have "bad genes." Once geneticists have identified target genes, it may be possible to treat cardiovascular problems with gene therapy or even to engineer the next generation of children so that heart disease is eradicated. Are we ready for this step?

A slightly more futuristic scenario involves nanotechnology—the construction of microscopic devices capable of performing delicate tasks such as scraping clean the insides of clogged-up blood vessels and repairing damaged heart muscle. In a way, this seems fitting: A natural "machine" as remarkable as your heart deserves a team of ultra-high-technology mechanics to help to maintain its astounding level of performance.

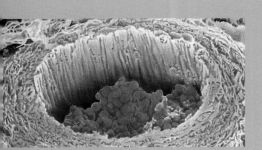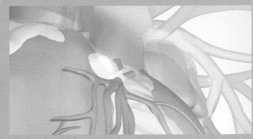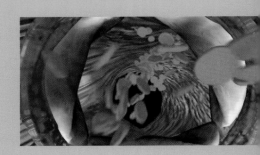

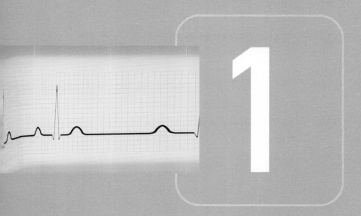

1

How your heart works

Your amazing heart and circulatory system

Your heart is a powerful "pump" that drives blood through the blood vessels, a vast "plumbing" network that stretches into every corner of your body. Together, pump and plumbing make up your cardiovascular system.

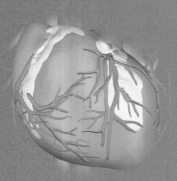

YOUR BODY'S LIFELINE

Blood provides your body's cells with the vital nutrients they need to survive and function, but unless it can be transported around the body and delivered to where it is needed, it is useless. Your cardiovascular system ("cardio" = heart; "vascular" = blood vessel) provides this capability.

A journey through the system

Over the following pages, we examine how the heart looks from the outside and inside, explaining the unique elements that enable it to fulfil its demanding role, including the cardiac muscle that pumps the blood, the electrical system that triggers muscle contraction, and the set of valves that direct the blood's flow. We look at the overall circulatory network and its major components, showing how they work together to deliver blood to each of the body's 75 trillion cells. We take you on an exciting visual journey through the heart from the perspective of a red blood cell, and we end by taking a look at the control mechanisms in the brain that coordinate the whole cardiovascular system.

Did you know that the heart undergoes radical structural change at the moment of birth—the only major organ of the body to do so? **For more information, see pages 34 to 35.**

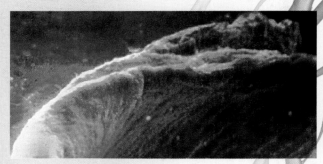

As simple as AVC
Blood vessels—arteries, veins, and capillaries—have different names depending on their size and whether they carry blood away from or toward the heart; *see pages 30 to 31.*

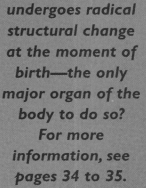

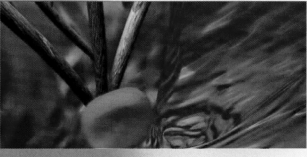

The ride of your life
How does it feel to be a red blood cell hurtling through your heart? *Turn to pages 32 to 33 for an insider's view of what you would see.*

Where is your heart?
Do you know exactly where your heart is in your chest? What would you see if you could open up your ribcage and take a look inside? Turn to pages 18 to 19 to find out.

Red or blue?
Blood vessels carrying oxygen-rich blood, such as arteries, are colored red. Veins, meanwhile, are shown in blue as they carry blood depleted of oxygen.

A double-sided structure
Your heart is divided into a left and a right side, and each of these sides is split into a top and bottom chamber. This simple, four-chamber organization enables maximum efficiency; see pages 20 to 21.

Amazing muscle power
Our lives depend on our unrelenting heartbeat, produced by the very special type of muscle in the heart. Find out what makes it unique and how it manages to go on and on . . . see pages 22 to 23.

Mirror image
Because the heart is usually shown as if you were looking at it from the front, features on the left side of the picture are actually on the right side of the heart, and vice versa.

The heart on the outside

The heart lies hidden beneath the shield of the breastbone, enveloped in a bag of lubricating fluid. Dozens of blood vessels course over its surface, supplying the fuel that powers the unrelenting motion of its muscular walls.

The aorta *is the body's largest artery. It rises up from the left side of the heart.*

The left lung

The left auricle *is a flap of muscle that is part of the left atrium; it inflates when filled with blood.*

The left coronary artery *is the main vessel supplying blood to the left side of the heart.*

Insulating fat *hides the groove that marks the border between the two lower chambers of the heart—the interventricular sulcus.*

The pericardium *envelops the heart and contains the lubricating pericardial fluid.*

The tip, or apex, *of the heart is the part nearest the front of the chest.*

A front view of the heart
Among the prominent features in this view of the outside of the heart are the coronary arteries and veins that stretch across the outside of the chambers, carrying the heart's own blood supply.

YOUR TWISTED HEART

The heart itself bears little resemblance to the symbol familiar from valentine cards and cartoons. It is a grapefruit-sized mass of muscle shaped like a cone with a blunt, rounded tip or apex. If you could peer inside your own chest, you would see that your heart does not sit square in the center—It is just to the left of the midline and is both tilted and twisted slightly, so that the apex is toward the front of the chest.

Your heart beats an amazing 100,000 times a day—That's 36 million times a year!

Well protected

Reflecting the massive importance of the heart to the functioning and survival of the body, evolution has buried it deep within the torso, in the most protected location possible. The heart lies beneath the hard, bony plate in the center of your chest—the breastbone or sternum; ribs on either side provide added protection. This bony cage overlies a "bag" containing the heart—the pericardium. This fibrous sac is filled with pericardial fluid, which both protects the heart and lubricates its constant motion.

Finding your heart

By following landmarks on your chest, you can locate the tip and top of your heart. Run your fingers down the midline of your chest, there should be a ridge of bone just above nipple level. Move your finger a little to the left to feel your second rib. Between this and the next rib is a space, underneath which is the top of your heart. Count to the fifth space down, keeping close to the sternum. Imagine a line straight down from the center of your left collarbone, and then move your finger left until you meet it—women may have to lift the left breast to find this point. Your finger should now be over the tip of your heart, where it is closest to the skin.

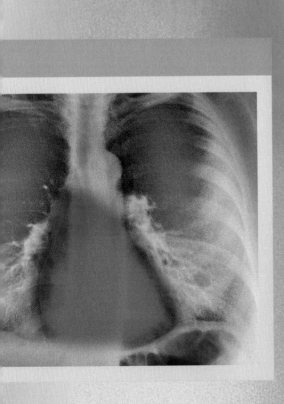

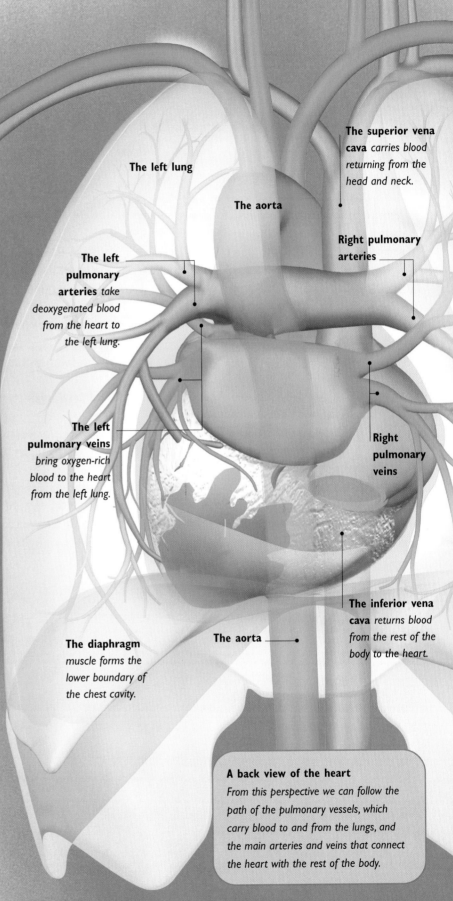

The left lung

The aorta

The superior vena cava *carries blood returning from the head and neck.*

Right pulmonary arteries

The left pulmonary arteries *take deoxygenated blood from the heart to the left lung.*

Right pulmonary veins

The left pulmonary veins *bring oxygen-rich blood to the heart from the left lung.*

The diaphragm *muscle forms the lower boundary of the chest cavity.*

The aorta

The inferior vena cava *returns blood from the rest of the body to the heart.*

A back view of the heart
From this perspective we can follow the path of the pulmonary vessels, which carry blood to and from the lungs, and the main arteries and veins that connect the heart with the rest of the body.

Inside the heart

Like all the best and most reliable designs, the inside structure of the heart is simplicity itself. The organ is divided into two distinct sides—right and left—with an upper and lower chamber on each side.

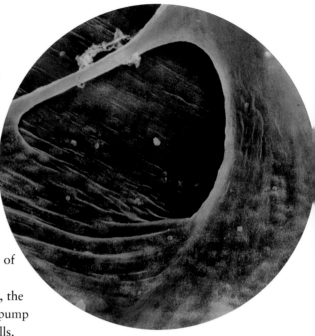

WHY DOES THE HEART HAVE TWO SIDES?

Having two sides allows the heart to keep blood that is depleted in oxygen separate from blood that is oxygen rich. By the time blood returns to the heart after its journey around the body, its oxygen content is low and needs to be refreshed. The heart collects this low-oxygen blood in its right-hand chambers and then drives it toward the lungs to pick up oxygen. The oxygen-rich blood returns to the left side of the heart, which pumps it out to the body.

The two sides are not directly linked—there is a thick wall of muscle, the septum, between them. Nor are they symmetrical—the left side has to pump blood much further than the right, so it has thicker, more muscular walls.

WHY ARE THERE UPPER AND LOWER CHAMBERS?

Each side of the heart has an upper chamber, the atrium (plural: atria) and a lower chamber, the ventricle. This division makes the heart more efficient at collecting and pumping out blood. Blood entering the heart collects in the atria, which then squeeze it into the ventricles. When full, the ventricles contract to force the blood out toward the lungs or the rest of the body.

Because the atria have to push blood only to the next chamber, they have thin walls, making them relatively small chambers. The ventricles are bigger, with thick walls of muscle, as they need to work much harder.

An inside view
This electron micrograph shows the internal surface of a ventricle. Small red blood cells on the surface are just visible, as is a papillary muscle projecting from the ventricle wall.

Separating the upper and lower "decks"

The heart is built around a framework of tough, fibrous material, which forms a plate, or "fibrous skeleton," between the upper and the lower chambers of the heart. This plate provides an anchor point for the heart's hard-working valves (see pages 26 to 27) and also acts as an insulation barrier to prevent electrical impulses in the upper chambers from triggering premature action in the lower chambers (see pages 24 to 25).

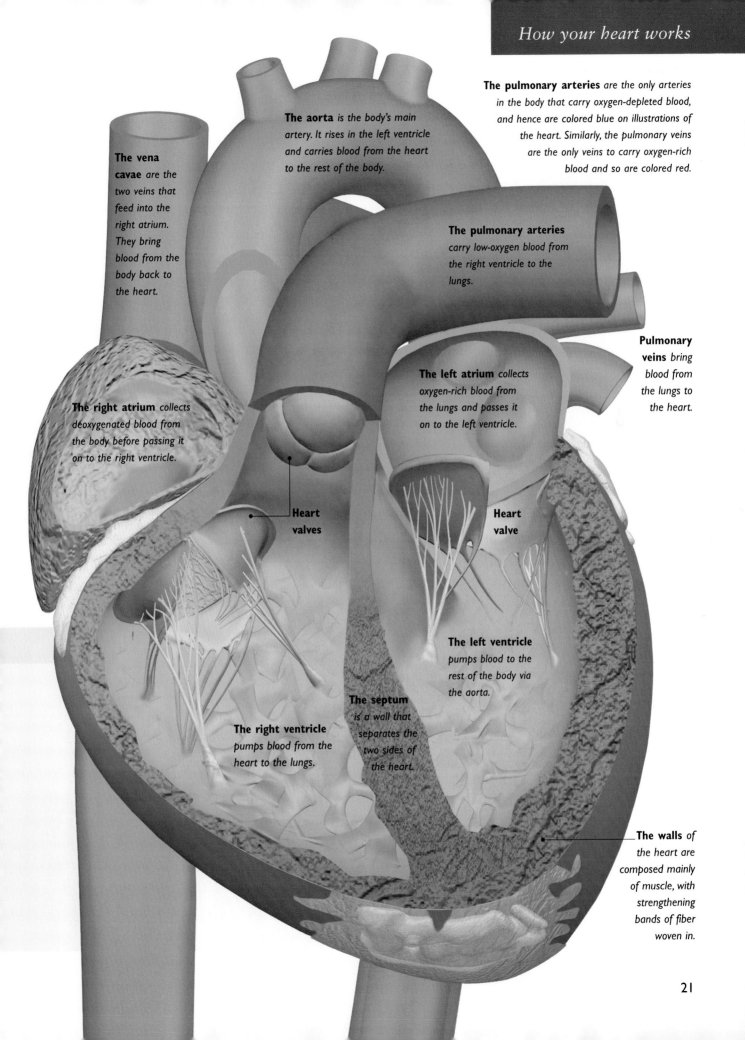

The vena cavae *are the two veins that feed into the right atrium. They bring blood from the body back to the heart.*

The aorta *is the body's main artery. It rises in the left ventricle and carries blood from the heart to the rest of the body.*

The pulmonary arteries *are the only arteries in the body that carry oxygen-depleted blood, and hence are colored blue on illustrations of the heart. Similarly, the pulmonary veins are the only veins to carry oxygen-rich blood and so are colored red.*

The pulmonary arteries *carry low-oxygen blood from the right ventricle to the lungs.*

Pulmonary veins *bring blood from the lungs to the heart.*

The right atrium *collects deoxygenated blood from the body before passing it on to the right ventricle.*

The left atrium *collects oxygen-rich blood from the lungs and passes it on to the left ventricle.*

Heart valves

Heart valve

The left ventricle *pumps blood to the rest of the body via the aorta.*

The septum *is a wall that separates the two sides of the heart.*

The right ventricle *pumps blood from the heart to the lungs.*

The walls *of the heart are composed mainly of muscle, with strengthening bands of fiber woven in.*

21

The heart muscle

Heart muscle is a remarkable tissue, with unique properties that allow it to perform astonishing feats of performance and endurance. It is able to meet these demands because of special adaptations that set it apart from ordinary muscle.

BETTER BY DESIGN

The demands placed on your heart muscle fibers far exceed those made on the toughest machines built by humans. These fibers must contract and relax in perfect concert more than once a second, without rest, every single day of your life. In times of stress or physical exertion, their workload can rise by up to 300 percent, and they must not fail, or the rest of the body cannot function. So, heart muscle fibers contain many structures called mitochondria—the energy-producing "generators" that power each cell in your body; they also hold extensive energy reserves. Each fiber is cross-linked to others all around it to increase their collective strength and power.

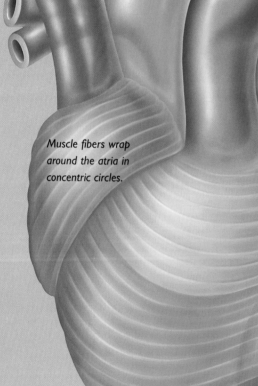

Muscle fibers wrap around the atria in concentric circles.

Layer upon layer of muscle fibers spiral around the ventricles.

The main squeeze

When the signal to contract travels through the fibers of the atrial walls, they squeeze the blood down into the ventricles. When the signal passes through the ventricular fibers, they contract in a wringing motion, squeezing the blood out from the bottom upward— similar to rolling up a tube of toothpaste at the same time as squeezing it.

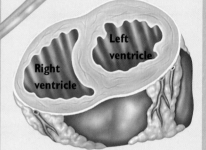

In a relaxed state

Thick . . .
The thick muscular walls of the left ventricle can create enough pressure to pump blood around the whole body.

. . . and thin
The right ventricle has less of a distance to pump blood—just to the lungs—so its walls are less muscular.

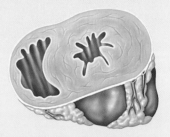

During contraction

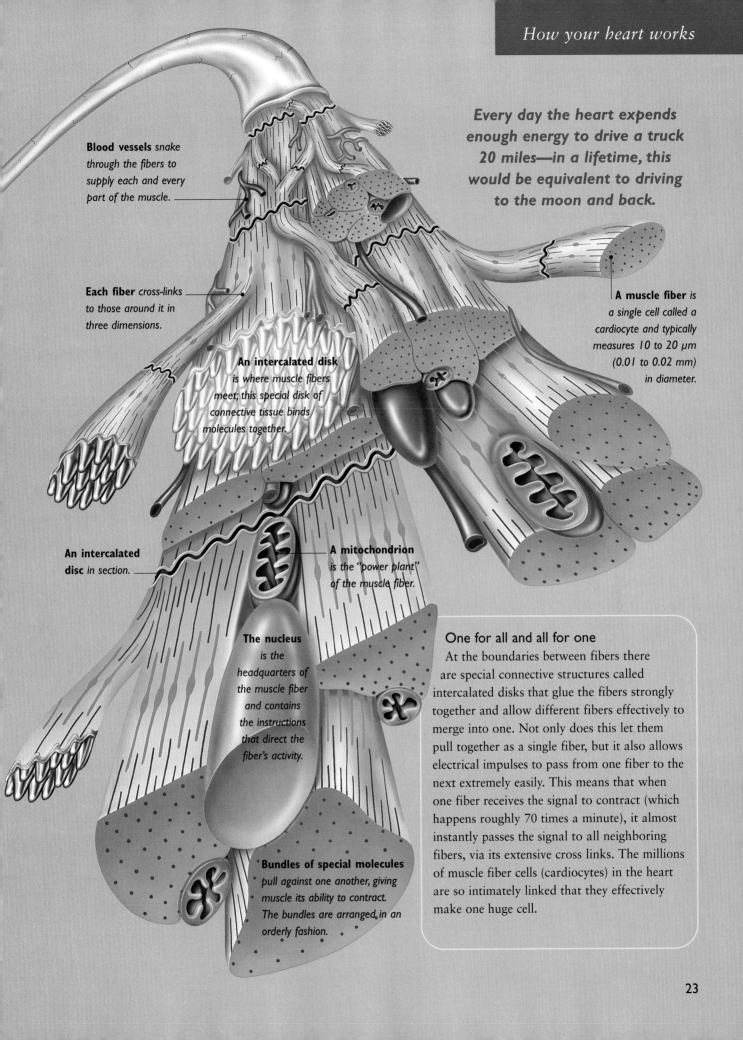

Blood vessels *snake through the fibers to supply each and every part of the muscle.*

Every day the heart expends enough energy to drive a truck 20 miles—in a lifetime, this would be equivalent to driving to the moon and back.

Each fiber *cross-links to those around it in three dimensions.*

A muscle fiber *is a single cell called a cardiocyte and typically measures 10 to 20 μm (0.01 to 0.02 mm) in diameter.*

An intercalated disk *is where muscle fibers meet; this special disk of connective tissue binds molecules together.*

An intercalated disc *in section.*

A mitochondrion *is the "power plant" of the muscle fiber.*

The nucleus *is the headquarters of the muscle fiber and contains the instructions that direct the fiber's activity.*

Bundles of special molecules *pull against one another, giving muscle its ability to contract. The bundles are arranged in an orderly fashion.*

One for all and all for one

At the boundaries between fibers there are special connective structures called intercalated disks that glue the fibers strongly together and allow different fibers effectively to merge into one. Not only does this let them pull together as a single fiber, but it also allows electrical impulses to pass from one fiber to the next extremely easily. This means that when one fiber receives the signal to contract (which happens roughly 70 times a minute), it almost instantly passes the signal to all neighboring fibers, via its extensive cross links. The millions of muscle fiber cells (cardiocytes) in the heart are so intimately linked that they effectively make one huge cell.

The heart's electrical conduction system

The heart beat is automatically generated by the heart's own electrical impulses. Each impulse sets off a sequence of heart muscle contractions that is coordinated to the millisecond by special fibers within the heart.

R The big spike—the QRS complex—represents the electricity in the ventricles making them contract.

The initial hump, the P-wave, represents electrical signals traveling through the atria.

The T-wave reflects the ventricles relaxing.

SETTING THE PACE

The different chambers of the heart must contract in precise sequence to send the blood on its journey around the body. This sequence is triggered by the heart's natural pacemaker—the sinoatrial node—and coordinated by a unique system of wiring. Here we take you through the electrical cycle of one heartbeat, showing how it relates to an ECG trace.

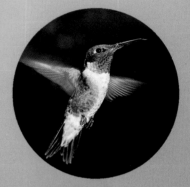

Poetry in motion
The process of signal generation and conduction takes just 200 milliseconds (0.2 sec). It is over in a blink of an eye, yet in that time a hummingbird will have flapped its wings four times.

The sinoatrial node *is the cardiac pacemaker.*

The atrioventricular node *sits between the upper (atria) and lower chambers (ventricles) and relays the signals to the ventricles.*

The bundle of His, *also known as the atrioventricular bundle, carries the signal to the Purkinje fibers.*

Purkinje fibers *radiate out within the heart's muscle to stimulate ventricular contraction.*

24

After each beat, there is a pause as the sinoatrial node recharges before the next contraction.

P

Because the heart supplies its own electrical impulses, it can continue to beat even when separated from the body, as long as it has an adequate supply of oxygen and nutrients.

1 The sinoatrial node generates electrical signals at regular intervals. Conducting fibers carry the signal from this node to the atrioventricular node. At the same time, the signal spreads out and passes through the walls of both atria, which contract and squeeze blood into the ventricles. The fibrous ring that lies between the atria and the ventricles insulates the upper and lower chambers.

R

Q S

2 At the atrioventricular node, the impulse is boosted and sent down a thick bunch of conduction fibers in the wall between the two ventricles. This bunch—the bundle of His—immediately splits into two "bundle branches," which fan out across the inside walls of the ventricles.

R

T

Q S

3 The bundle branches deliver the signal to the Purkinje cells, which spread out as fibers in the ventricle walls. Starting from the lower tip of the heart, the signal to contract passes from muscle fiber to muscle fiber, triggering a wave of contraction that spreads upward.

4 The ventricles relax and the sinoatrial node "recharges," so it is ready to fire and start the sequence again. Any disturbances to this coordinated sequence result in arrhythmias, which doctors can detect using an electrocardiogram (ECG).

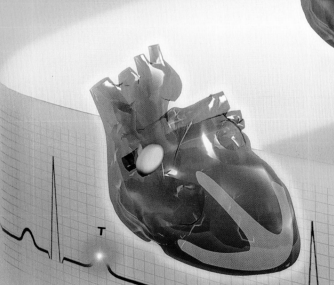

T

The heart's valves

Keeping huge quantities of blood flowing around the body in the right direction every second of the day and night is a formidable task. To meet this challenge, the heart employs a unique set of four valves.

The familiar "lubb-dupp" sound of your own heart beating is made by the pairs of valves slapping shut.

ASTOUNDING FEATS OF NATURAL ENGINEERING

The heart has four valves—the tricuspid and mitral, which control the flow of blood between the atria and the ventricles within the heart, and the pulmonary and aortic valves, which control blood flow between the heart and the rest of the body. Each valve opens and closes some 36 million times a year, with precise split-second timing; the whole cycle takes less than a second. Thin and lightweight yet fantastically durable and reliable, the valves are superb examples of engineering that far outperform anything devised by scientists.

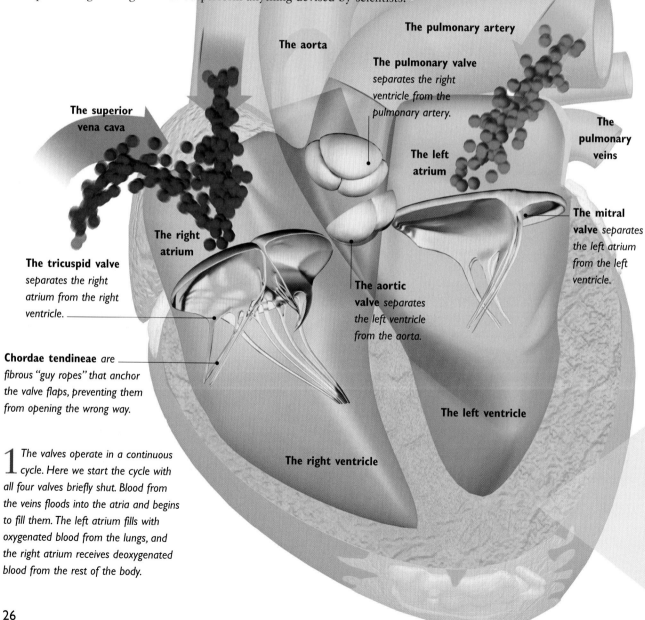

The aorta

The pulmonary artery

The pulmonary valve *separates the right ventricle from the pulmonary artery.*

The superior vena cava

The left atrium

The pulmonary veins

The mitral valve *separates the left atrium from the left ventricle.*

The right atrium

The tricuspid valve *separates the right atrium from the right ventricle.*

The aortic valve *separates the left ventricle from the aorta.*

Chordae tendineae *are fibrous "guy ropes" that anchor the valve flaps, preventing them from opening the wrong way.*

The left ventricle

The right ventricle

1 *The valves operate in a continuous cycle. Here we start the cycle with all four valves briefly shut. Blood from the veins floods into the atria and begins to fill them. The left atrium fills with oxygenated blood from the lungs, and the right atrium receives deoxygenated blood from the rest of the body.*

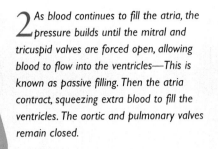

2 As blood continues to fill the atria, the pressure builds until the mitral and tricuspid valves are forced open, allowing blood to flow into the ventricles—This is known as passive filling. Then the atria contract, squeezing extra blood to fill the ventricles. The aortic and pulmonary valves remain closed.

3 Pressure builds in the ventricles as they fill up and falls in the atria as they empty of blood. This change in pressure causes the mitral and tricuspid valves to snap shut, preventing back flow of blood into the atria. The ventricle walls now start to contract and pressure in the ventricles soars.

4 The ventricles continue to contract, forcing a surge of blood at massive pressure toward the aortic and pulmonary valves. These valves open in response to the pressure and force of the blood: The deoxygenated blood in the right ventricle passes into the pulmonary artery on its way to the lungs, while the oxygenated blood in the left ventricle goes out through the aorta to the rest of the body. As the surge subsides and the ventricles relax, the valves close to prevent blood flowing back into the heart.

The circulatory system

The total length of all the blood vessels in your body is around 60,000 miles—enough to go around the Earth more than twice. Together these vessels make up the circulatory system of your body.

Even when you are resting, it takes just over 1 minute for all 8 pints of your blood to be pumped around your body.

THE CIRCLE OF LIFE

Your blood carries the oxygen and nutrients that you need to function and survive, but it requires a delivery system to help it reach each of the thousands of billions of cells in your body. At the center of the system is your heart. Large vessels called arteries carry blood away from here, branching repeatedly to create smaller arteries—several hundred of them. After the blood has passed through the various tissues of the body, it is taken back to the heart by vessels called veins. Hundreds of small veins merge to create progressively larger ones, bringing the blood back to the heart.

Move along now

How does blood get from the heart, around the body, and back to the heart again? The circulatory system has built-in features designed to do just that.

Artery

Vein

The heart drives blood into the arteries at high pressure (indicated by the size of the arrows).

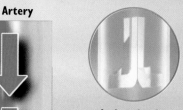

A closed valve
Valves in veins snap shut to prevent backflow of blood.

The arteries' walls are elastic and muscular, which helps to maintain this pressure.

Open valves *allow blood through.*

Veins rely on internal valves as well as the squeezing action of muscles around them to propel low-pressure blood back to the heart.

As arteries branch into successively smaller vessels, the pressure falls off, as it spreads out over a large surface area.

People who have to stand for long periods, such as soldiers and surgeons, can suffer dizziness as blood starts to pool in the lower portions of the body. To avoid this, they flex their calf muscles to pump blood up from their legs.

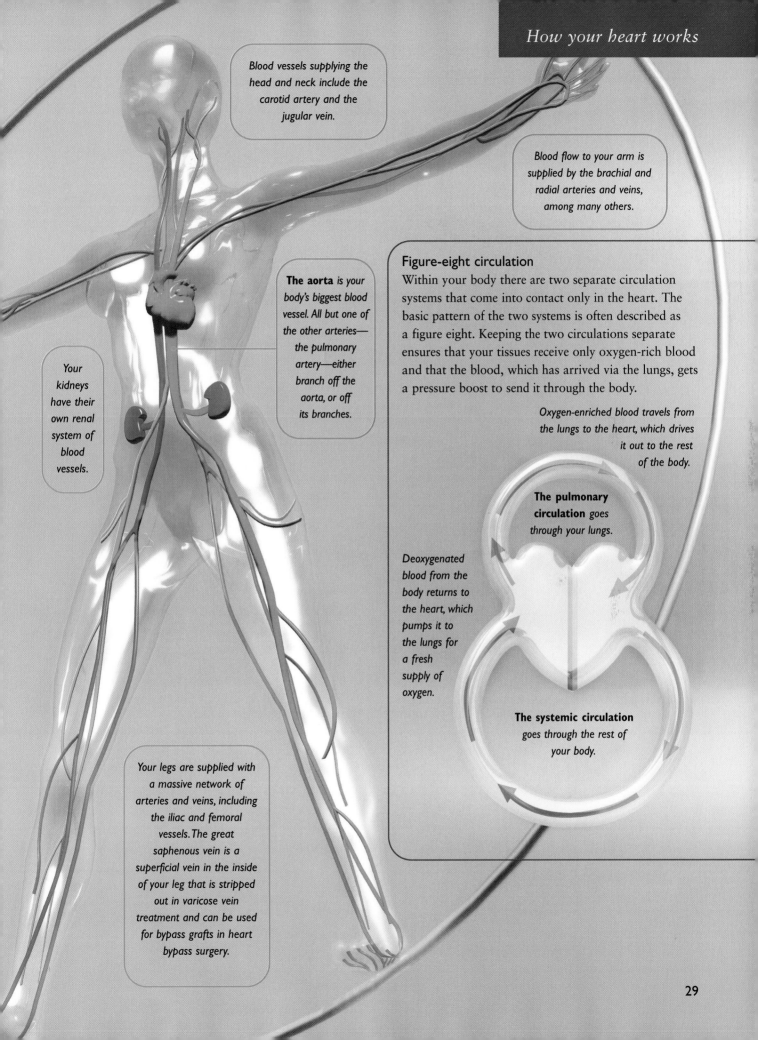

Blood vessels supplying the head and neck include the carotid artery and the jugular vein.

Blood flow to your arm is supplied by the brachial and radial arteries and veins, among many others.

The aorta *is your body's biggest blood vessel. All but one of the other arteries— the pulmonary artery—either branch off the aorta, or off its branches.*

Your kidneys have their own renal system of blood vessels.

Figure-eight circulation

Within your body there are two separate circulation systems that come into contact only in the heart. The basic pattern of the two systems is often described as a figure eight. Keeping the two circulations separate ensures that your tissues receive only oxygen-rich blood and that the blood, which has arrived via the lungs, gets a pressure boost to send it through the body.

Oxygen-enriched blood travels from the lungs to the heart, which drives it out to the rest of the body.

The pulmonary circulation *goes through your lungs.*

Deoxygenated blood from the body returns to the heart, which pumps it to the lungs for a fresh supply of oxygen.

The systemic circulation *goes through the rest of your body.*

Your legs are supplied with a massive network of arteries and veins, including the iliac and femoral vessels. The great saphenous vein is a superficial vein in the inside of your leg that is stripped out in varicose vein treatment and can be used for bypass grafts in heart bypass surgery.

29

Arteries and veins

The circulatory system is made up of five basic kinds of blood vessels. Some are large enough to carry quarts of blood every minute; others are so small that only one blood cell at a time can pass through.

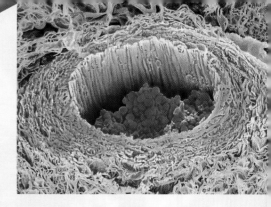

An arteriole in section
Tiny red blood cells can be seen traveling through the lumen of this arteriole, colored pink, sitting within connective tissue.

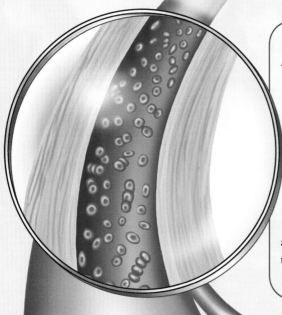

Arteries

As large vessels with thick, highly elastic, muscular walls, arteries help the heart to move blood around the body by doing some squeezing of their own. Waves of contraction travel along the biggest arteries, carefully timed to boost the heart's own pumping efforts. The elastic walls of arteries help them to maintain the high blood pressure that drives blood around the body.

An arteriole *is a smaller vessel that branches off an artery, and then branches several times itself.*

An artery *is a large vessel that is the primary supplier of blood to a whole body area.*

The middle layer of the artery contains concentric sheets of smooth muscle.

The innermost layer includes abundant elastic fibers and a lining called the endothelium.

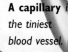

A capillary *is the tiniest blood vessel.*

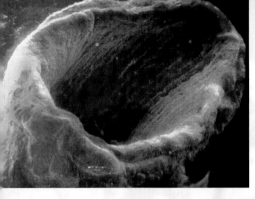

A vein in section
In comparison with the arteriole (left), the wall of this vein is much slimmer and more flaccid, due to having less muscle and more elastic fibers.

Veins

Although they may be as wide as arteries, veins do not have to deal with such high blood pressures. As a result they have much thinner walls, with fewer elastic and muscle fibers. This structure means that veins are more easily flattened by the movements of surrounding muscles than muscular arteries are. Veins have one-way valves to keep blood flowing toward the heart and to prevent it from going back the other way (see page 28).

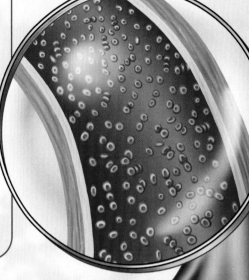

A venule *is a smaller vein—the average diameter is 0.02 millimeter.*

A vein *results from merging smaller venules and carries the oxygen-depleted blood back towards the heart.*

The capillary bed *is a dense network of capillaries.*

If you opened up all the capillaries in an adult body and laid them out flat, the total surface area of the walls would be about two-thirds that of a football field.

The middle muscular layer is the same thickness as the inner elastic layer.

The internal surface of the vein is made up of an inner elastic layer covered by an endothelial lining.

Capillaries

There are millions of these tiny vessels in your body; often they are no wider than a single red blood cell (less than 0.001 mm), and their walls may be just one cell thick. Pores and gaps in these walls allow the free flow of substances back and forth between the blood and the target tissues outside the capillary, letting nutrients out and waste products in.

A complete cardiac cycle

A typical red blood cell passes through the heart more than 1,200 times in a day and is subjected to great pressures for fractions of a second. Join us on a rollercoaster ride through the heart, seeing the action from the red cell's point of view.

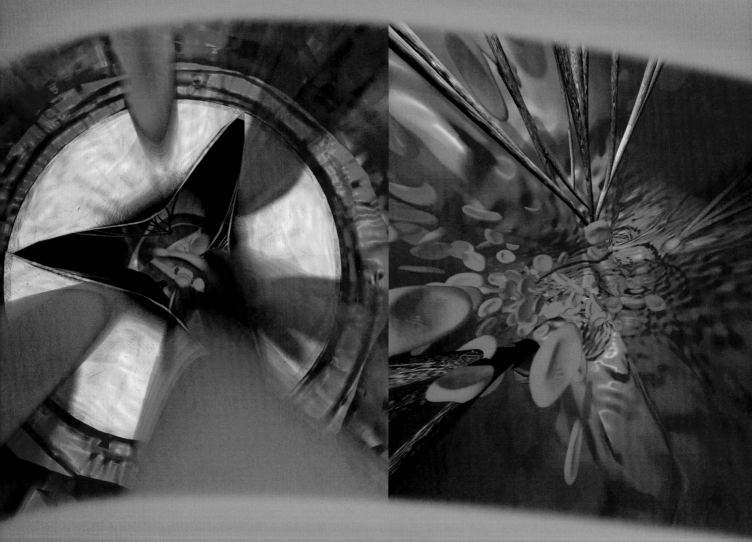

All aboard
The heart is relaxed and filling up with blood from around the body. The tricuspid valve (between the right atrium and the right ventricle) opens and blood flows through. The pacemaker cells have just fired and a wave of electrical activity spreads through the atrial walls. The ride is about to begin. Our red blood cell has just arrived, depleted of oxygen, in the right atrium, and is traveling toward the right ventricle.

Changing rooms
In response to the electrical signal, the walls of the right atrium squeeze our red cell into the right ventricle at top speed. The same thing is happening simultaneously on the left side of the heart: The contracting atria force blood into the ventricles in addition to passive filling. Meanwhile, the electrical signal passes down the septum: When it reaches the apex, the Purkinje cells will distribute it through the ventricle walls.

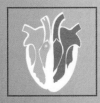

To the lungs

As the electrical signal passes through the muscle fibers, they contract. The ventricle walls close in with extreme force. First, the tricuspid and mitral valves slam shut; then, the pulmonary and aortic valves fly open. With a sudden surge the blood cell rushes out of the heart and up the pulmonary artery toward the lungs. The heart itself has just completed a single beat, but our red cell is only halfway through its cardiac ride.

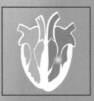

Back to the heart—then beyond

After a whistlestop tour of the lungs to pick up oxygen, the red cell reaches the left atrium, where a new phase of atrial contraction helps it on its way into the left ventricle. The new impulse triggers another wave of muscle contraction, and the rising pressure of the plasma fluid—in which the cell floats—forces the mitral valve shut, closing the route from the atrium. Soon the pressure will force the aortic valve open and speed our cell into the aorta to start its journey round the body.

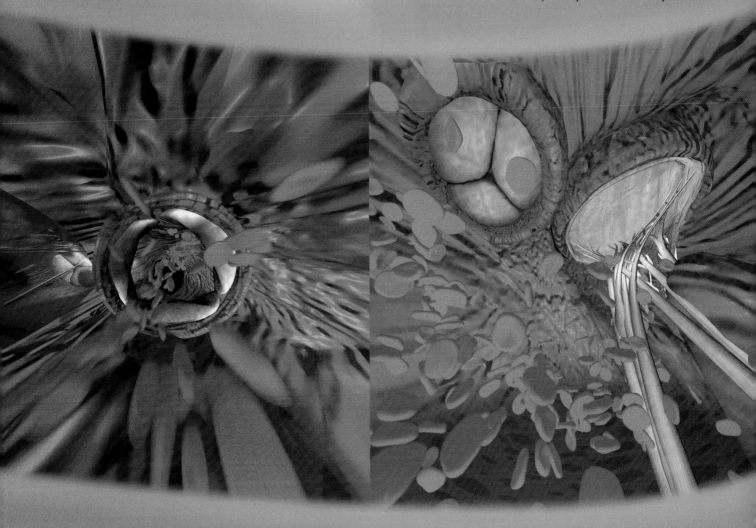

Over 75 trillion cells throughout your body rely on your heart to keep them supplied with oxygen and nutrients.

Get inside the action
These computer-generated images, based on detailed anatomy of the heart, present a unique view of the heart's inner workings.

How the heart changes at birth

The heart is unique among your body's organs in that it undergoes major anatomical changes at birth. Blood flow is radically redirected, to equip the newborn baby for life outside the womb.

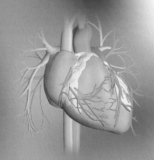

UMBILICAL CIRCULATION

Unborn babies have some major blood vessels that we all lose after our birth—the umbilical arteries and vein. A baby in the womb depends on its mother's placenta to supply oxygen and nutrients (which we get by breathing and eating) and to remove waste products (which we exhale or excrete). Within the umbilical cord, two umbilical arteries take deoxygenated blood from arteries in the baby's legs to the mother's placenta, while a single umbilical vein delivers nutrient- and oxygen-rich blood directly to the baby's liver. From there, the fresh blood flows through a vein called the ductus venosus into the vena cava, which feeds it into the right side of the heart, before starting its journey around the body.

On diversion—the blood's route through the unborn heart

Because a baby in the womb does not breathe and fill its lungs with oxygen, there is no point in sending blood there to pick up its oxygen supply. Instead, the baby gets all the oxygen-rich blood it needs from its mother, and its heart employs circulatory shortcuts, rather like temporary traffic diversions, to redirect the blood more efficiently. Most people have heard of the condition called "a hole in the heart." Few realize, however, that we were all hole-in-the-heart babies until we took our first breath. To reduce blood flow to the nonfunctioning lungs, unborn babies have a hole, called the foramen ovale, in the wall between the left and right atria. This hole allows a lot of the blood in the right atrium to pass directly to the left atrium, bypassing the right ventricle and lungs. Another shortcut, the ductus arteriosus, allows blood to pass from the pulmonary artery straight into the aorta. When you took your first breath, your lungs inflated and the two shortcuts very quickly closed up. In some babies, however, this does not happen properly, and the holes remain open. Today, the holes can be closed by surgery to enable the heart to function normally.

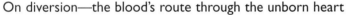

Ductus arteriosus

Foramen ovale

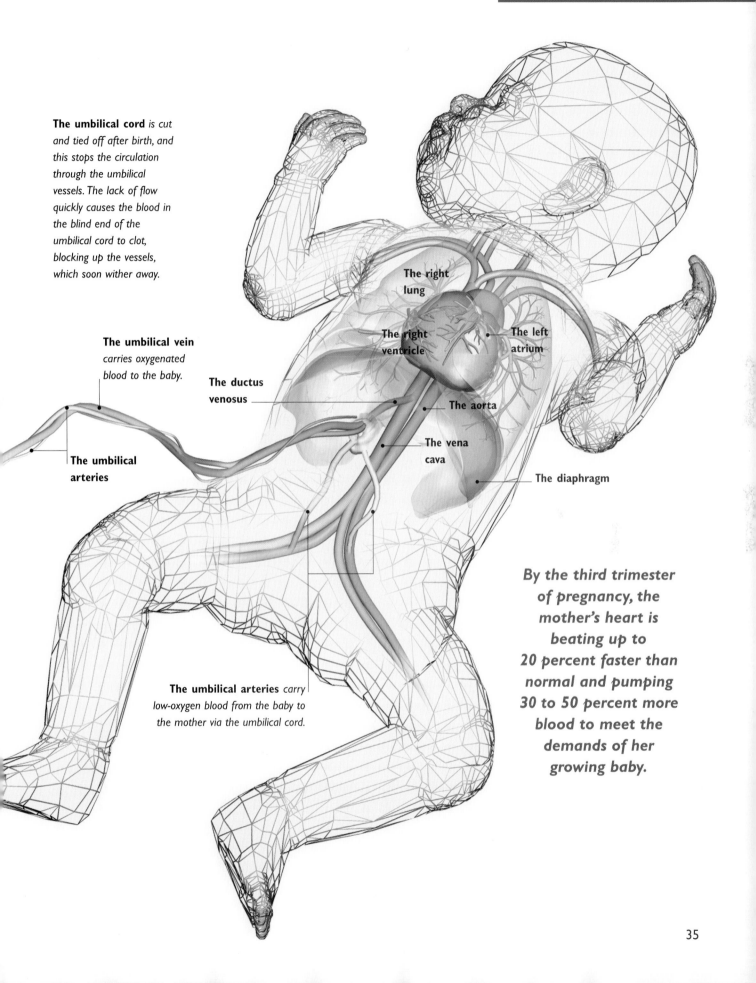

The umbilical cord *is cut and tied off after birth, and this stops the circulation through the umbilical vessels. The lack of flow quickly causes the blood in the blind end of the umbilical cord to clot, blocking up the vessels, which soon wither away.*

The umbilical vein *carries oxygenated blood to the baby.*

The ductus venosus

The umbilical arteries

The right lung

The right ventricle

The left atrium

The aorta

The vena cava

The diaphragm

The umbilical arteries *carry low-oxygen blood from the baby to the mother via the umbilical cord.*

By the third trimester of pregnancy, the mother's heart is beating up to 20 percent faster than normal and pumping 30 to 50 percent more blood to meet the demands of her growing baby.

A day in the life of your heart

Your heart has to adjust its rate and output to respond to the demands of varying activities. Control centers in your brain monitor the heart's performance and send signals that change the rate at which it beats at a moment's notice.

CONTROL CENTERS

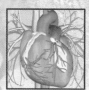

An area of the brain stem called the medulla contains centers that control your heart and circulation—the cardiovascular centers. They receive information from receptors in your blood vessels and the heart: Chemoreceptors are sensitive to concentrations of gases dissolved in the blood, such as oxygen and carbon dioxide; baroreceptors measure blood pressure. These centers operate as two halves: One relays messages to the heart via the cardiac nerve to make the heart speed up (excitatory); the other sends signals via the vagus nerve to slow the heart down (cardioinhibitory).

In addition to controlling heart rate, these centers determine how much blood flows to different parts of the body. At rest, for example, the muscles receive about 1 pint per minute, but when you exercise, the cardiovascular centers divert blood from other organs, increasing the supply to your muscles to as much as 30 pints per minute.

If the heart's pacemaker was left to its own devices, it would make the heart beat about 100 times a minute. When you are at rest, however, signals received via the vagus nerve constantly inhibit the heart, slowing it down to a normal rate of around 70 beats per minute.

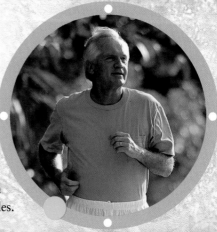

7:00 A.M. Early morning run

It's early in the morning, your heart rate is slow, and your muscles relaxed. What better way to get you going than a jog through the neighborhood? As you start to exercise, you increase the rate at which your muscles burn glucose for energy. Chemoreceptors in your arteries detect rising levels of carbon dioxide from the working muscles, indicating that your heart needs to work harder to send the muscles extra oxygen-rich blood. The cardiovascular centers receive this information and send signals down the cardiac nerve to increase heart rate and the strength of the heart's contractions, and to divert extra blood to the muscles.

11:30 P.M. Bedtime

Sleep gives your body a chance to rest. As your consciousness shuts down, your body switches into low gear. Reduced muscle activity means that less glucose is burned. Oxygen in the blood is not used up at the same rate, and less carbon dioxide is produced. The cardiovascular centers receive this information from the chemoreceptors and slow the heart down via the vagus nerve, which inhibits the pacemaker cells, causing them to produce fewer impulses. Thus, your resting body can save energy, allowing your heart to take it easier for a while.

6:30 P.M. Traveling home

On the way home in your car, you are forced to make an emergency stop. As you slam on the brakes, your pulse is racing, your blood pressure soars, and you can feel your heart pounding. These responses are part of the fight-or-flight mechanism, which is initiated by the shock. Epinephrine is released into the bloodstream and binds to receptors on your heart, speeding up your heart rate to prepare you for action. After a couple of minutes, your pulse and blood pressure return to normal.

1:00 P.M. Big lunch

At last it is time to eat. As you fill up on food, stretch receptors in your stomach and chemoreceptors in your intestines stimulate the cardiovascular centers, via the hypothalamus. This reinforces the process of redirecting blood to your digestive system.

12:30 P.M. It must be lunchtime

The smell of food cooking gets your mouth watering and, more important, triggers a part of the brain called the hypothalamus. This activates your cardiovascular centers, which signal various blood vessels around the body to direct blood toward the intestines and liver, where it is needed to help them pick up nutrients from your lunch.

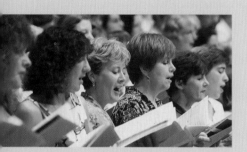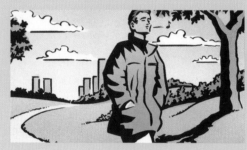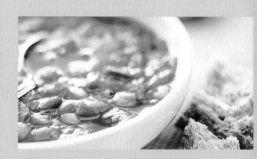

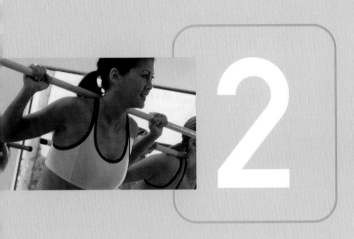

2

Heart-healthy living

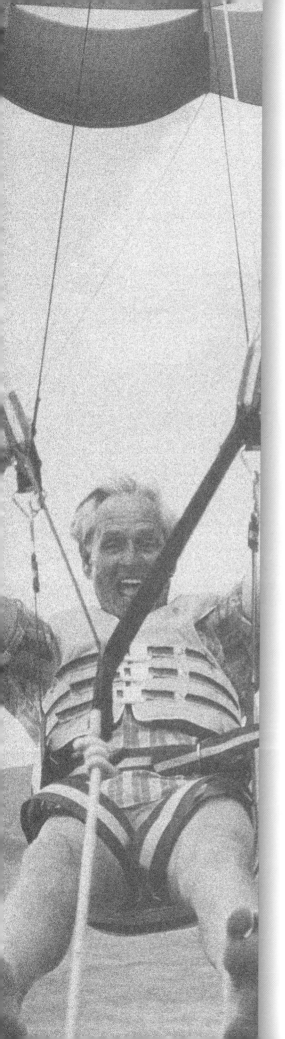

TAKE CHARGE OF YOUR HEART HEALTH

There's now a wealth of information on what makes for a healthy heart, so don't leave your heart health to chance. Brush up on your knowledge of factors that increase your risk of heart disease. Then, if you have to, take measures to avoid them. Work with your doctor and make sure you have screening tests—such as those for blood pressure and cholesterol—when you need them.

 41

Are you at risk for heart disease? Find out what the risks are—and what you can do to avoid them and safeguard your heart health.

 48

Learn to become self-aware and to look out for warning signs of heart disease.

Take responsibility for your health

The health of your heart is very much in your hands. By understanding the various risk factors that influence your cardiovascular health, you can help to safeguard the future of your heart and circulatory system.

Why do some people suffer from heart disease while others live a lifetime free of cardiovascular complications? Sometimes it may seem as though heart health is a lottery, but in practice we know a lot about what influences the chances of developing heart or circulatory problems. Such knowledge is extremely valuable because it greatly increases our ability to identify our risk of heart disease. Once we have identified factors in our lifestyles that may put us at risk, we can take measures to change them.

HEART RISK FACTORS

So what does influence your cardiovascular prospects? Decades of research have uncovered a range of factors that contribute to the development of heart and circulatory problems. These factors may not cause cardiovascular disease directly, but they do increase its likelihood— hence, they are known as risk factors. There are two types of risk factor— those you can't do anything about and those that can be modified, either by changes in lifestyle or by medical intervention.

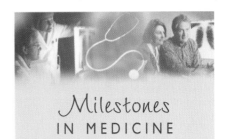

Milestones
IN MEDICINE

In 1948, the U.S. government established the Framingham Heart Study. A sample of 5,029 adults living in Framingham, Massachusetts, were selected and their health has been followed ever since. The study has helped to identify and assess risk factors and how they interact. The data obtained from the study form much of the basis of the current approach to heart disease.

Adding up your risk factors for heart disease

First, find the box that matches your age, sex and smoking status. Next, find your blood pressure and blood cholesterol:HDL ratio (see page 46 for more information on cholesterol measurement). Use the color in the corresponding cell to find your risk of a heart attack or stroke in the next five years.

Risk of cardiovascular "event" in five years

| 0–5% | 10–15% | 20–30% |
| 5–10% | 15–20% | |

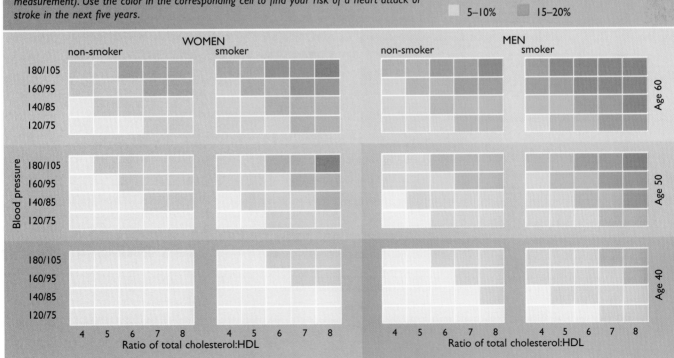

Unmodifiable risk factors

The main factors that you cannot control include the following:

- **Age** This is one of the biggest risk factors for heart disease—The older you are, the greater the risk. More than half of those who have heart attacks are over 65.
- **Gender** Men are much more likely than women to develop conditions linked with narrowing of the arteries, at least until age 65. This increased risk is thought to be attributable to the influence of hormones, which are protective in women until menopause.
- **Genes** Heredity plays a part in almost all illnesses and certainly affects the health and longevity of your cardiovascular system. A history of cardiovascular disease in your family is therefore a major risk factor for your own health.
- **Race** Some racial groups seem to be at higher risk of cardiovascular problems. African-American men,

IT'S NOT TRUE!

"Good genes protect you from CAD"

Coronary artery disease (CAD) is less common in certain parts of Africa and Asia than in Western countries. But the low rate of CAD is probably due to external factors such as diet rather than an innate genetic factor. People who move to the West and adopt a Western lifestyle show the same rate of CAD as the indigenous populations of their new countries.

Crystals of estrogen
After menopause, when levels of the hormone estrogen plummet, the risk of heart disease in women begins to increase.

for instance, are much more likely to suffer from high blood pressure.

- **Diabetes mellitus** This condition significantly increases the risk of coronary artery disease and stroke.

All these factors are beyond your control, but it is important to be aware of them, nonetheless. Knowing that you belong to a risk group gives you the chance to work harder on those factors that you can control and helps to alert your healthcare providers to potential warning signs, so that problems can be identified and treated early.

Modifiable risk factors

There are many serious influences on your cardiovascular health that you can control wholly or in part.

- **High blood pressure** This is a particularly significant risk factor for stroke, but also for other cardiovascular illnesses.
- **High blood-cholesterol levels** These are strongly linked to narrowing of the arteries, which in turn causes or exacerbates many other cardiovascular conditions. Blood cholesterol levels 20 percent above the norm can double the risk of a heart attack.
- **Smoking** Between 30 and 40 percent of deaths from coronary artery disease can be attributed to smoking. It is the main risk factor for sudden cardiac death.
- **Obesity** Being overweight is linked to poor heart health, and those who are obese—more than 30 percent over ideal body weight—are

particularly at risk. Obese women in the 30 to 55 age group, for instance, have three times the risk of heart disease of women who are a healthy weight.

- **Stress** Constant stress may be damaging to your general health and could increase the risk of heart attack, although there is little scientific evidence to support this.

On the following pages we survey some of these factors in more detail, starting with a look at some gender- and age-related issues—factors that you cannot change or control—then focusing on those factors that can be modified or avoided.

MEN VERSUS WOMEN

On average, women live six years longer than men, a difference attributable in large part to lower rates of heart disease. Although this picture is slowly changing as women now smoke in numbers comparable to men, it seems clear that women enjoy some level of biological protection against cardiovascular disease. Hormones seem to be key, and their importance is indicated by the changes in women's heart health following menopause.

Hormones and the heart

During menopause, hormonal changes occur that have a major impact on a woman's risk of cardiovascular disease. Menopause usually occurs at around 45 to 55 years of age and is associated with a dramatic fall in the levels of estrogen and progestogen.

High estrogen levels before menopause mean women have lower blood pressure, less obesity, lower "bad" LDL cholesterol and higher "good" HDL cholesterol than men—reducing the risk of heart disease. Following menopause, this protective effect is lost, and obesity, cholesterol, and blood pressure levels gradually increase until they are higher than those in men by age 65. The incidence of coronary artery disease consequently increases until, by about age 75, it has caught up with men. The overall effect of oestrogen on the heart, therefore, is to delay the onset of coronary artery disease in women by about 10 years.

By following the guidelines for improved cardiovascular health—adopting a healthy lifestyle, eating a balanced diet, and exercising more —

Before menopause, women's risk of coronary artery disease is half that of men, but smoking 30 cigarettes a day removes much of that benefit.

you can help to offset the negative cardiovascular effects of menopause on your heart health.

HRT under pressure

Hormone replacement therapy (HRT) seems to improve levels of blood cholesterol, but its overall beneficial effect on the heart and circulation may have been over-estimated; in some cases, taking HRT after the menopause can increase the risk of clot formation in the veins. Concerns exist that HRT may increase the risk of stroke, raised blood pressure, and cancer; these issues are the subject of current research.

If you already have high blood pressure, this should be controlled before commencing hormone replacement, but it doesn't mean you won't be able to take HRT. Talk to your doctor about the best combination of hormone therapy and blood pressure management for your particular condition.

BLOOD PRESSURE

High blood pressure, or hypertension, is a massive problem in developed countries. In the United States alone about 23 percent of the population is being treated for hypertension. It is a major risk factor for cardiovascular disease, although fortunately there are plenty of things that can be done to improve this condition.

First, however, you need to know your current blood pressure and what it means to your health.

Blood pressure changes

Your blood pressure fluctuates through the day—at its lowest during sleep, it rises on getting up and reaches its normal rate mid-morning. Woven into this pattern are times of excitement, nervousness, and activity—all of which raise blood pressure.

Systolic pressure

Diastolic pressure

Blood pressure (mmHg)

190

140

90

40

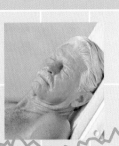

While you are asleep your blood pressure is at its lowest point—on average about 100/65 mmHg.

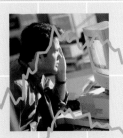

Stress and anxiety can cause blood pressure to shoot up as high as 190/115 mmHg.

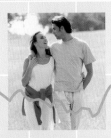

Standing or walking keeps a healthy adult's blood pressure at 120/80 mmHg.

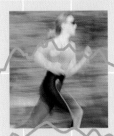

As you run, your heart beats faster, and blood pressure rises to about 160/105 mmHg.

Daily activity

Monitoring blood pressure during pregnancy

Your circulatory system undergoes enormous changes during pregnancy—blood volume, for example, can increase by as much as 40 percent. The pressure itself can either fall or rise, but usually diastolic pressure falls during the first and second trimesters by 10 to 20 mmHg, before increasing to prepregnancy levels by the time of delivery. A rise in blood pressure can be dangerous to both you and your baby, so your blood pressure will be measured at every prenatal checkup. This monitoring is especially important if you already had high blood pressure before your pregnancy. High blood pressure during pregnancy can damage the fetus and restrict its

growth in the uterus. It is also associated with preeclampsia and eclampsia—conditions that can be life-threatening for you and your baby. Regular monitoring of blood pressure means that appropriate action can be taken to prevent any serious consequences.

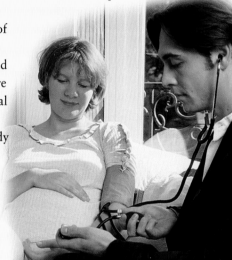

your heart is relaxing and filling up with blood. The two are expressed together—For example, the normal level of about 120/80 mmHg means a systolic pressure of 120 mmHg and a diastolic pressure of 80 mmHg.

The risk of cardiovascular disease rises with the level of blood pressure. People with high blood pressure can reduce this risk by lowering the pressure by making lifestyle changes and taking medication.

The combined results of more than 17 studies, which involved the treatment of more than 50,000 people with high blood pressure, showed the value of even small decreases in blood pressure. An average drop of just 5 to 6 mmHg in diastolic blood pressure over a five-year period reduced the number of strokes by one third, and the number of heart attacks was reduced by 16 percent.

Up and down

Your blood pressure varies with the time of day, the position of your body, your environment and activity, and how stressed you are. Blood pressure is controlled by the body's own feedback systems to within fairly narrow limits to prevent it from falling too much—Blood flow to the organs, especially the brain, is reduced if blood pressure drops too much. Although a temporary rise in blood pressure is normal in some situations—such as during exercise— sustained high pressure causes damage to the heart, which can lead to heart failure and an increased risk of atherosclerosis and strokes.

Blood pressure increases with age in most populations in the developed world. However, research suggests that

the rise is not inevitable and probably reflects the cumulative impact on the circulatory system of high salt consumption, low fruit and vegetable intake, obesity, and lack of exercise.

Measuring pressure

Blood pressure is measured with a device called a sphygmomanometer. This device uses a column of mercury to measure pressure—Blood pressure readings are therefore given in millimeters of mercury (mmHg in scientific notation). Two readings are taken: The first—systolic pressure— shows the pressure while your heart is squeezing and pumping blood into the arteries so that it exerts maximum force on the walls of your blood vessels; the second—diastolic pressure—shows the pressure while

Getting it checked

You should have your blood pressure checked by your doctor every five years until at least age 75. If your blood pressure is more than 140/90 mmHg, the doctor will want to repeat the check to confirm that it is high and to make a decision about treatment. If you need treatment, your doctor will want you to have your blood pressure measured regularly until it has fallen to a healthy level. If your blood pressure is only slightly elevated and you are otherwise well, you may not need to take medication, but you will need to be monitored regularly.

White-coat hypertension

Some people have high blood pressure readings when they are in a doctor's office, but their readings are normal at other times. Although the person may not be aware of it, the stress of being in the doctor's office temporarily raises his or her blood pressure. This phenomenon is known as white-coat hypertension.

In general, doctors believe that this kind of short-lived episode of high blood pressure does not require treatment. One of the best methods of identifying white-coat hypertension is to have a 24-hour ambulatory blood pressure monitor. This involves being fitted with a portable monitor that reads and records your blood pressure as you go about your daily business, allowing your doctor to measure your blood pressure in situations that reflect your normal environment.

THE CHOLESTEROL STORY

The health of your heart and circulatory system are closely related to the levels of cholesterol in your body. The details of how and why are complex, involving a battery of technical names such as HDL and LDL cholesterol and triglycerides. These terms refer to fatty substances, called lipids, in your blood. The two most important types of lipid, in terms of the health of your arteries, are cholesterol and triglycerides.

Cholesterol finds its way into your body from your diet but is also manufactured by the liver. It is used by your body to maintain cell structure. Almost all foods contain some cholesterol, but particularly rich sources include eggs, red meat, liver, and shrimp and other shellfish.

Triglycerides is the collective term for the saturated and unsaturated fats that you hear about in reference to food. These fats are an important energy source for your body and are particularly abundant in meat and

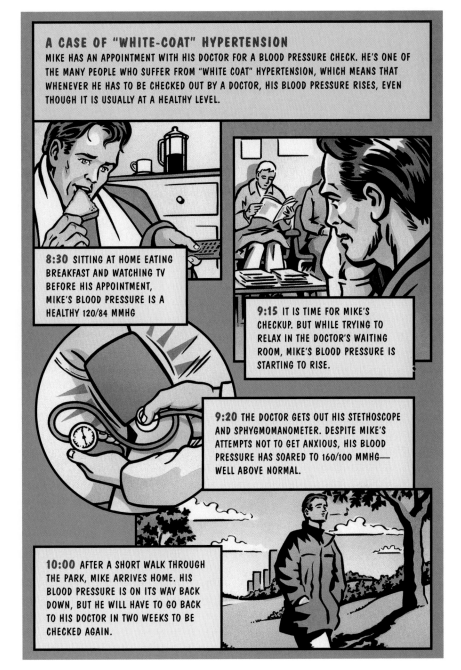

A CASE OF "WHITE-COAT" HYPERTENSION
MIKE HAS AN APPOINTMENT WITH HIS DOCTOR FOR A BLOOD PRESSURE CHECK. HE'S ONE OF THE MANY PEOPLE WHO SUFFER FROM "WHITE COAT" HYPERTENSION, WHICH MEANS THAT WHENEVER HE HAS TO BE CHECKED OUT BY A DOCTOR, HIS BLOOD PRESSURE RISES, EVEN THOUGH IT IS USUALLY AT A HEALTHY LEVEL.

8:30 SITTING AT HOME EATING BREAKFAST AND WATCHING TV BEFORE HIS APPOINTMENT, MIKE'S BLOOD PRESSURE IS A HEALTHY 120/84 MMHG

9:15 IT IS TIME FOR MIKE'S CHECKUP. BUT WHILE TRYING TO RELAX IN THE DOCTOR'S WAITING ROOM, MIKE'S BLOOD PRESSURE IS STARTING TO RISE.

9:20 THE DOCTOR GETS OUT HIS STETHOSCOPE AND SPHYGMOMANOMETER. DESPITE MIKE'S ATTEMPTS NOT TO GET ANXIOUS, HIS BLOOD PRESSURE HAS SOARED TO 160/100 MMHG— WELL ABOVE NORMAL.

10:00 AFTER A SHORT WALK THROUGH THE PARK, MIKE ARRIVES HOME. HIS BLOOD PRESSURE IS ON ITS WAY BACK DOWN, BUT HE WILL HAVE TO GO BACK TO HIS DOCTOR IN TWO WEEKS TO BE CHECKED AGAIN.

dairy products. Triglycerides appear to have similar effects on the health of the heart and circulatory system to those of cholesterol.

The effects of cholesterol

Although it has important biological functions, cholesterol can also be an extremely unhealthy substance. It has a major role in the development of

cardiovascular disease, the majority of which is caused by the build-up of cholesterol and other damaging material on the walls of arteries. This build-up, known as atherosclerosis, results in the narrowing of arteries, which can then lead to heart attacks and strokes because of a slowing or complete blockage of blood supply to part of the heart or brain.

BLOOD LIPIDS AND HEART HEALTH

Lipids are like oil—they do not dissolve in water or blood. In your body, lipids, including cholesterol and triglycerides, are transported in blood inside tiny "containers" called lipoproteins. There are two types of lipoprotein important to cardio-vascular health: HDL and LDL. LDL is know as "bad" cholesterol it increases the deposition of cholesterol in artery walls. HDL picks up cholesterol from around your body and takes it to the liver for disposal. Raised levels of HDL cholesterol counteract some of the detrimental effects of high LDL cholesterol: The object of a healthy diet is to lower your LDL levels while raising HDL levels.

Cholesterol globules

Of all the blood lipids, cholesterol is probably the best known. Cholesterol is insoluble in blood and is carried in containers called lipoproteins.

Triglycerides

Very high levels of triglycerides are toxic to the body, but there is little convincing evidence that they cause heart disease. There is evidence that high triglyceride levels are linked to low levels of HDL cholesterol, however, making them a risk factor.

How often should you have your cholesterol levels checked?

If you are fit and healthy, you will not need to have your lipid profile checked until age 40 if you are male, or until after the onset of menopause if you are female. Thereafter, unless your lipid profile is unfavorable, you only need to have it checked every five years. If you are diabetic, suffer from high blood pressure, or already have heart disease, you should have your blood lipids checked once a year.

If your lipid profile is poor and requires cholesterol-lowering drug treatment, you will be monitored until your levels are in a healthy range.

WHAT DOES YOUR CHOLESTEROL LEVEL MEAN?

Your lipid profile test gives you your total blood cholesterol level. Healthy and risky average levels of cholesterol have been established (see below). But age, blood pressure, and smoking habit must also be taken into consideration to get an accurate picture of your risk of cardio-vascular disease.

High risk > 117 mg/dL

Moderate risk 97 to 117 mg/dL

Lower risk < 97 mg/dL

Home or over-the-counter tests for cholesterol are available, but the results may not be as accurate as a sample analyzed in a professional laboratory, and interpretation is not always straightforward, so they are probably best avoided.

HAVING YOUR LIPIDS CHECKED

Measurements of cholesterol, triglycerides, and related lipids are combined to give your lipid profile— a snapshot of the types and amounts of lipids circulating in your blood. Your profile gives you your HDL:LDL ratio as well as your total cholesterol level.

Lipid profile report

These cholesterol and triglyceride levels are high, whereas HDL is low. Mr. Smith will have to make some dietary changes and possibly begin taking lipid-lowering drugs.

DEPARTMENT OF CHEMICAL PATHOLOGY PLEASANTVILLE HOSPITAL		Tel (914)222 2222 Fax (914)222-2223		
Address for report Dr. John Doe 11 Medical St. Pleasantville	Name F. C. Smith			
	Hospital No. 1234		Sex Male	D.o.B 7/17/47
	NHS No. 34567abc			
Consultant	Clinical Note			Lab No.

Cholesterol 113.4 mg/dL   (72—127.8)
Triglycerides 89.46 mg/dL   (9.0—37.8)
            Triglyceride reference range only
            valid for fasting samples
HDL Cholesterol 13.7 mg/dL   (14.4—25.2)
LDL Cholesterol LDL Cholesterol invalid due to high
            triglyceride concentration

Cholesterol: HDL ratio 8.3

Sample Date and Time 10/17/00	Investigation FASTING LIPIDS	Date reported 10/17/00

Low cholesterol = low risk

In parts of the world where average levels of cholesterol are low, such as in rural China, people experience less coronary artery disease than in areas with higher levels, such as the United States. Within these high-cholesterol populations, the risk of developing coronary artery disease relates directly to the level of blood cholesterol, with higher levels associated with higher risk.

The overwhelming message from health experts today is this: Keep your overall cholesterol level low. The lower it is, the lower your risk of developing heart disease. Lowering cholesterol with diet and drugs in high-risk people can reduce the development of coronary artery disease by as much as 40 percent.

ANTI-CORONARY-DISEASE LIFESTYLE

Studies of populations throughout the world show that high levels of heart and other arterial diseases reflect an unhealthy lifestyle. The rewards of living an anti-coronary-disease lifestyle are potentially huge—It will help you reduce your risk of developing high blood pressure, high cholesterol levels, and diabetes, and, if you already have any of these conditions, it will help you to treat them. In some cases it may prevent the need for, or reduce the amount of, prescribed medication.

Do not fall into the trap of thinking that you're too young to begin to be concerned about heart problems. Atherosclerosis takes years, even decades, before it causes symptoms. The beginnings of coronary artery disease can start to appear in your early twenties, so the sooner you make beneficial changes to your lifestyle, the better.

No smoking

Smoking is without doubt the most important preventable risk factor for cardiovascular disease. Deaths from cardiovascular problems increase by 18 percent in men and by 31 percent in women for every 10 cigarettes smoked per day. Stopping smoking halves the risk of developing cardiovascular disease within two to three years. See page 62 for more advice about giving up.

Eating right

The traditional Western diet typically contains an excess of saturated fats, cholesterol, and refined carbohydrates. Too much of these foods can lead to increased blood cholesterol, risk of obesity, high blood pressure and diabetes. A healthy diet has been proven to lower the risk of developing cardiovascular disease and to prevent recurrent problems in people with coronary artery disease. We take a detailed look at heart-healthy eating on pages 66 to 72.

Get fit and into shape

Regular physical activity is associated with a lower risk of coronary artery disease. Exercising more will lower cholesterol levels and blood pressure, improve your circulation, and help you to lose weight (see pages 80 to 81).

LEAD A HEART-HEALTHY LIFESTYLE

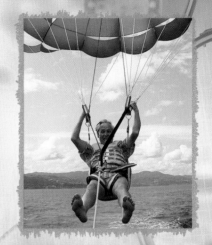

EXERCISE YOUR HEART *Exercise keeps you fit, and the benefits of exercise on the cardiovascular system are well proven.*

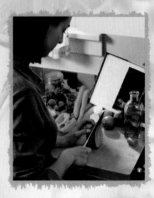

HEART-HEALTHY FOOD *Fruit and vegetables tip the scales in favor of less fat and more fiber, and reduce the risk of heart disease.*

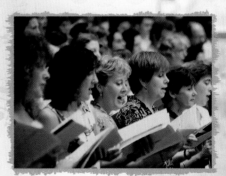

DON'T SMOKE *Smoking is the biggest risk factor for heart disease (see pages 60 to 63). Give up the habit and enjoy the greater capacity of your heart and lungs.*

Be involved in your health care

Your doctor can be more than just a port of call when you're ill: He or she can give you valuable advice for a healthy lifestyle. Learn to become self-aware and use your doctor wisely for a healthy heart throughout life.

Staying in shape has a lot to do with learning about your own body, and knowing what is normal and what is not. If you see that something is not quite right, write down some details about it: when it occurred, how long it lasted, and what, if anything, made it worse or better. Use the "Help your doctor to help you" boxes throughout this book to help focus on information that will be useful for your doctor in making a diagnosis.

WORKING WITH YOUR GP
We don't have much contact with our doctors after infancy, when checks for normal development are made, unless we are ill. But when we reach middle age or join a new doctor's practice, we are often invited for regular checkups, so that any problems can be picked up early and treated.

Take a proactive approach to your relationship with your doctor; know how often you should have your blood pressure checked, for example, or when your next cholesterol test is due. Arrange to have a full checkup, including tests for cholesterol, blood pressure, and diabetes, if not annually, then when you are approaching the age of 40 to 45 years if you are a man, or following menopause if you are a woman. Thereafter, if all is well, you should aim to have checkups at least every three to five years. If you are identified as being at high risk, checkups will need to be more frequent.

Be prepared
When you visit your doctor for a check-up, prepare beforehand to get the most from a consultation. Be ready to answer questions on symptoms or family history clearly. Read up on health issues related to the heart so that you know what the issues are. Work with your doctor to make sure that you get the maximum heart health benefits.

Regular is best
If you have been healthy all your life, you may find it difficult to fall into a routine of regular doctor's appointments when you reach middle age.

Get your blood pressure checked
Having a cardiovascular checkup enables your doctor to pick up problems early and start any needed treatment.

Get the go-ahead
In terms of heart health, exercise is very important, and everyone should be encouraged to give the heart a regular workout. If you begin a new sport, however, you need to consider your existing level of fitness and decide if the activity is suitable for you. Before embarking on a new exercise regime, make an appointment with your doctor to discuss any medical problems, and any age-related consider-ations, and to gauge your level of fitness. In this way, you and your doctor can agree a heart-safe exercise program that you can begin with confidence.

The need to discuss changes in your lifestyle may seem unnecessary, particularly if you have been very active, but think positively. Keeping up contact with your doctor is not a sign of physical weakness or impend-ing illness, but shows that you respect your body and want to keep it healthy now and in the future.

WATCH OUT FOR WARNING SIGNS
Being aware of suspicious symptoms, such as chest pain and breathlessness, allows early recognition of disease and can improve the effectiveness of treatments. Not all chest pain is heart related, so don't panic the minute you experience discomfort. Talk to your doctor, who can decide whether your symptoms indicate something serious.

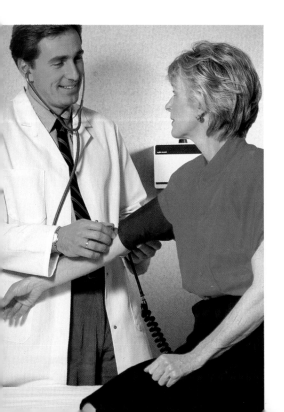

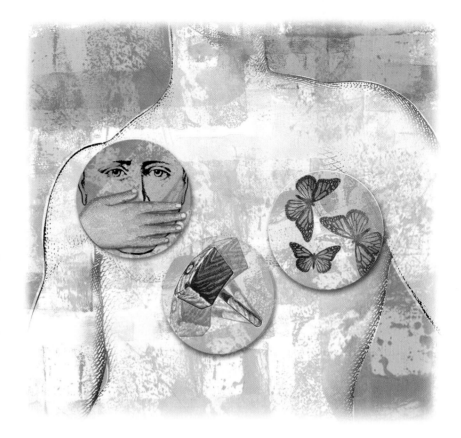

Do you experience chest pain?

The most common symptom associated with the heart is chest pain, also known as angina. Characteristically, angina is felt as a pain or discomfort in the center of the chest. Sometimes, this pain travels up into the neck and jaw, or down the left arm.

Words that are often used to describe the pain of angina include "tightness," "constriction," "pressure," "weight," or "ache." Angina doesn't vary with breathing, movement, or position, and pressing on the chest will not make the pain worse.

The pattern of the symptoms is also important. Angina pain is brought on by exercise, emotion, and stress and is relieved by rest. Consult your doctor if you are at all concerned about any discomfort or pain in your chest.

Do you get breathless?

A second major symptom of heart trouble is shortness of breath. Although there are many other causes, shortness of breath can be associated with angina or heart failure. The shortness of breath may only occur on exertion, but if the damage to the heart is more severe, it may not pump properly even at rest, and fluid can build up in the lungs, making it difficult to breathe. People with heart failure often feel breathless when they are lying flat in bed and have to prop themselves up on pillows. They may also wake in the middle of the night because of

difficulty breathing. In some people, these symptoms are accompanied by swelling of the ankles and legs. This collection of symptoms is highly suggestive of a heart problem and merits urgent medical attention.

A fluttering in the chest?

Palpitations, the sensation of your heart beating, does not automatically result from a heart condition; it can be brought on by too much strong coffee. But palpitations can be a

symptom of a heart rhythm problem—arrhythmia—especially if you feel dizzy or have blackouts. If in doubt, consult your doctor.

Do you have poor circulation?

Pain in the joints, such as the knees, hips, and ankles, is common and suggests a condition such as arthritis. Pain in the calves, thighs, or buttocks that occurs during exertion, however, could indicate peripheral vascular disease, in which the arteries in the

Healthy teeth, healthy heart

Having a good dental routine can protect you not only against gum disease and tooth decay but may also influence the risk of heart disease. People with poor oral health may be more likely to have atherosclerosis—clogging up of the arteries—which can precipitate a heart attack. Some experts believe the bacteria that accumulate in the gums and teeth enter the bloodstream and affect blood clotting. People who have defective heart valves are at particular risk of endocarditis—infection of the valves.

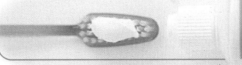

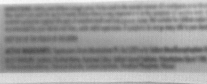

In a normal day, the contraction and relaxation of muscles in the legs help blood to return to the heart. If you have to spend a long period sitting down—during a long flight or an all-day car trip, for example—your risk of developing potentially dangerous blood clots in your leg veins rises because of a pooling of blood in the veins. A few simple measures can help prevent this from happening.

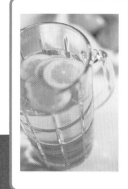

Drink plenty of water. Dehydration increases the likelihood of clots. Keeping up your intake of fluids is essential; ensure that you avoid alcohol, as this is a diuretic and will cause you to lose more fluid.

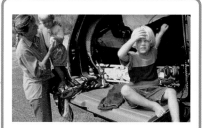

Stretch your legs. Stop regularly during long car rides and get out of the car; if you are traveling by plane, get up and walk around every two hours.

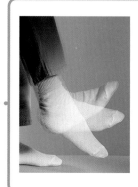

Point and flex your feet. If you can't leave your seat, exercise your leg muscles (to boost blood returning to the heart) by flexing and pointing your feet. Use the floor as resistance.

Should everyone take an aspirin a day?

In cases of coronary or carotid artery disease, doctors advise a daily dose of 75 mg of aspirin—equivalent to one children's aspirin or half a normal tablet. Aspirin thins the blood and so reduces the risk of heart attack and stroke. Some people with high blood pressure, which puts them at higher risk of cardiovascular disease, also benefit from a low dose of aspirin daily. Consult your doctor first before starting to take aspirin regularly, though, because it can cause side effects such as stomach problems and ulcers.

ASK THE EXPERT

legs become narrowed by atherosclerosis and the blood supply to the muscles can be inadequate.

The brain has a very good blood supply from four arteries that pass up the neck. If one of these arteries is gradually blocked, the blood supply to the brain is maintained from the other arteries. But if clots of blood travel to the brain, they may cause a sudden blockage and impair brain function, either temporarily or permanently (stroke). Symptoms such as a sudden weakness of part or the whole of one side of the body, or loss of the ability to speak for a few minutes, need urgent attention.

MEDICINES AND YOUR HEART

Some of the medicines in use today have side effects that impact heart health, although usually the benefits of prescribed drugs outweigh these potential risks. Significant risk of heart damage is small with daily medications. Some tricyclic antidepressants alter heart rhythm, and arrhythmias can also, rarely, be associated with certain antihistamines. If you are concerned about any potential side effects of medicines, talk to your doctor.

On the pill

The oral contraceptive pill is a very safe, reliable form of contraception; but it does have some risks. Women who take the pill have a higher risk of blood clots in the legs, brain, and, to a lesser extent, the arteries of the heart. The risk, however, is small: if 250,000 women take the pill for one year, it will cause on average only one stroke. But the risks associated with pill use rise considerably if you smoke, have high blood pressure, or if you are over the age of 35.

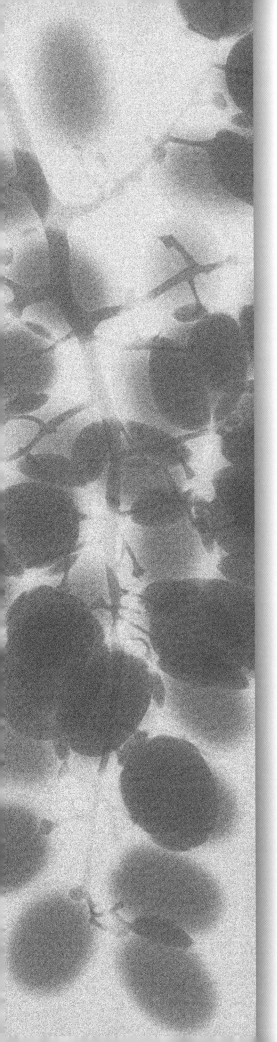

ADOPT A HEART-HEALTHY LIFESTYLE

So many aspects of life can have an impact on the health of your heart and circulatory system—some of them detrimental, others beneficial—but it's never too late to adopt a heart-healthy lifestyle. Did you know that if you smoke, you can reduce your risk of a heart attack by half within five years by giving up? Or that having a glass or two of wine isn't going to harm your heart—it may even be of benefit? Use this section to find out if you need to change your lifestyle to take care of your heart.

52 *Stress can raise both blood pressure and cholesterol levels—major risk factors for heart disease—so learn how to handle it.*

54 *Sleep gives your heart a breather, allowing it to slow down and recuperate, so make sure you're getting enough.*

56 *A daily drink might be good for your heart, but don't overdo your alcohol consumption.*

60 *Smoking damages the heart directly and restricts blood flow to all parts of your body. Check out some tips to break the habit.*

64 *Keep tabs on your caffeine habit; it has some surprising effects on your heart and cardiovascular system.*

Taking charge of stress

If you have ever experienced a sudden scare, you will know the sensation of your heart thumping fast and loud in your ears. But what is really happening to your cardiovascular system in times of tension and when you are under pressure?

A pounding heart is one element of the body's innate fight-or-flight response to stress. The brain signals the adrenal glands to release the hormone epinephrine into the blood-stream, and this increases the rate and force of the heartbeat. The heart pumps faster to send blood to the brain and the muscles in preparation for attack or retreat. In isolated instances, the heart rate usually returns to normal within minutes, after the source of stress is gone. But what happens when the cause of stress is not short term? Does the cardiovascular system undergo continuous strain when we start a new job or lose a loved one? And

what about the sustained pressure of, for example, a high-powered career or even loneliness?

FEELING THE STRAIN

Stress affects two of the principal risk factors for the development of coronary heart disease—blood pressure and cholesterol. Studies have found that blood pressure and cholesterol levels rise in response to a variety of stresses, from arguments to video games. The immediate effects of stress, apart from the release of epinephrine and a racing heart, are to increase blood pressure and cholesterol levels, make the heart more susceptible to disturbances of rhythm, and cause platelets within the blood to bind more readily. Great emotional upset, such as the loss of a loved one, can cause angina in those with coronary artery disease; in some cases, sudden severe shock can precipitate a heart attack.

Under long-term stress, release of the natural steroid hormone cortisol increases, causing salt retention, a rise in blood volume and blood pressure, and a greater sensitivity to the action of epinephrine.

Blood pressure risks

The pressure of the blood circulating around your body needs to remain within a certain range in order for your heart to function healthily. When the pressure rises above a certain level—at a time of stress, for example—the heart has to work harder than normal. Like any

muscle, the heart muscle becomes strained with the sustained effort of working against the high pressure and may eventually weaken, leading to congestive heart failure. People

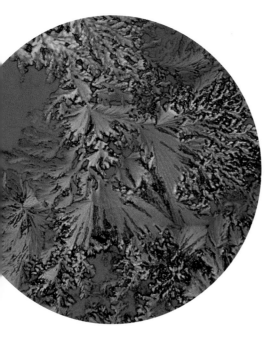

Chemical reaction
This colored microscopic photograph shows crystals of the hormone epinephrine, which prepares your body for "fight or flight."

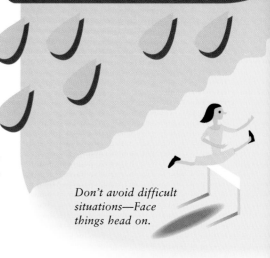

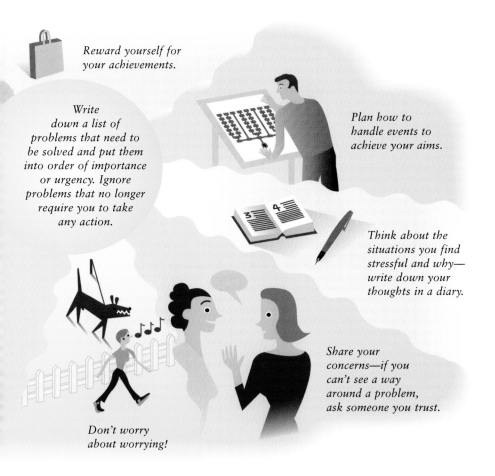

Reward yourself for your achievements.

Write down a list of problems that need to be solved and put them into order of importance or urgency. Ignore problems that no longer require you to take any action.

Plan how to handle events to achieve your aims.

Think about the situations you find stressful and why— write down your thoughts in a diary.

Share your concerns—if you can't see a way around a problem, ask someone you trust.

Don't worry about worrying!

Having palpitations

Blood pressure and heart rate are carefully tuned to meet the body's demands without conscious thought or perception. Sometimes, however, we are suddenly aware of our heart beating. When palpitations occur out of the blue, they can be very disturbing. Occasional palpitations are usually harmless, but you should consult your doctor if you are worried. Before your appointment, think about how you would answer the following questions.

- *When do you experience the palpitations? For example, do they usually follow a stressful event, or do they occur when you are lying in bed at night?*

- *Are the palpitations regular or irregular? Pay attention to the rhythm of your heartbeat. Your doctor may ask you to drum it with your finger.*

- *Do you have any other symptoms, such as faintness or dizziness?*

with uncontrolled high blood pressure are at least three times more likely to have coronary artery disease, six times more likely to have congestive heart failure, and seven times more likely to have a stroke than people whose blood pressure is controlled. There are no obvious symptoms of high blood pressure, so ask your doctor to monitor yours on a regular basis.

MANAGING STRESS

Some degree of stress is normal and can even improve your performance at certain tasks. For example, actors sometimes claim that the stage fright they suffer before going on stage gives an extra edge to their performance. But when anxiety becomes excessive, prolonged, or frequent, not only do you perform less efficiently, but you could also

suffer real mental and physical harm. It is vital to be aware of the danger signs and be prepared to take some action to manage your stress levels.

Reap the benefits of relaxation

You can learn a number of "coping" techniques to help you remedy the short-term effects of stress. Progressive relaxation is one simple way to reduce anxiety and muscle tension. First, tense and then relax each group of muscles in turn. At the same time, concentrate on deep, slow breathing, using the diaphragm rather than just the chest.

Another technique is biofeedback training. With this technique, you are presented with a stressful situation and your body's responses are then "fed back" auditorily or visually— using a beeping sound or a graph on a monitor. This technique is often

used to help people with high blood pressure. A sensitive cuff monitors blood pressure, and a sound is emitted when the pressure rises. The person must learn to stave off the sound by concentrating on relaxing and breathing to reduce the pressure.

Massage is another great technique for relaxation, and the sweeping strokes toward the heart may help improve blood flow and ease tension.

Sleep and the healthy heart

Sleep is an important time for your heart—taking things easier for a few hours gives it a vital chance to recharge. Insufficient rest can spell trouble for the cardiovascular system, particularly for people with heart problems.

Just as you need to recoup after a hard day's work, so does your heart. A good night's sleep is essential to provide a refreshing respite for your whole cardiovascular system. It allows your heart rate to fall and blood pressure to drop.

WHILE YOU WERE SLEEPING
Sleep requirements change with age. Over the age of 25, our ability to catch up on lost sleep by sleeping during the day or having a long "nap" greatly diminishes, probably

Night-time activity
Sleep is a time for recuperation and recovery from the day's activities, but it's not all rest. During the night we may move around many times and the heart rate changes accordingly.

because of changes in brainwave activity. As we grow older, we may find that we need less sleep, and may wake more often during the night. Fortunately, these natural alterations in sleep requirement do not appear to impact heart health.

In your dreams
Sleep time is divided into rapid eye movement (REM) sleep and non-REM sleep. During the non-REM stages of sleep—when we are sleeping deeply— the heart slows down to 40 to 50 beats a minute compared with a normal waking level of 60 to 80 beats a minute. During the REM stages—the time when we dream—the heart returns to a normal conscious rate. As you

imagine yourself moving about within your dreams, your heart behaves accordingly, speeding up when you dream you are running, for instance, or when you are in a stressful situation.

Getting enough sleep?
When you miss out on sleep, your cardiovascular system misses out on the benefits of relaxation. Prolonged lack of sleep can sometimes cause irregular "jumping" heartbeats called premature ventricular contractions (PVCs). In some cases, the person may even feel as though his or her heart has stopped briefly. PVCs are an example of "palpitations"—an awareness of the heart beating—and can also be caused by poor sleep. Although these can be worrisome, they are usually harmless, and all that is needed is a good night's sleep.

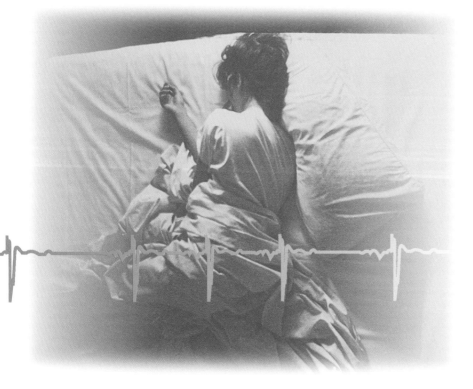

In some cases, however, there may be an underlying heart disorder, so visit your doctor if symptoms persist.

THE INSOMNIA PROBLEM

One in three Americans, or almost 100 million people, have trouble sleeping; one-third of them reported finding insomnia a chronic problem.

The most common cause of insomnia is probably stress, which can cause one to have difficulty falling asleep and staying asleep, or to wake too early. If insomnia is stress-related, it is usually resolved as the source of stress is tackled and overcome.

People who suffer from palpitations caused by lack of sleep can become trapped in a vicious cycle, with anxiety aggravating the insomnia. A few simple relaxation aids may help. For instance, as you lie in bed, breathe deeply and slowly, relax your muscles, and concentrate on slowing down your heart beat. Turn to the section on stress (page 53) for more relaxation tips.

SNORING AND THE HEART

Snoring is common and not usually a problem, but some heavy snorers may have the condition obstructive sleep apnea (OSA), which can affect the heart. Classically, OSA affects overweight, middle-aged men, although it can occur in other adults and in children with enlarged tonsils.

When someone suffering from OSA snores, the upper airways become sucked shut until the sufferer is woken by the struggle to breathe. If the gap between breaths is prolonged, there is a drop in the amount of oxygen in the blood and a reduction in heart rate. When momentary waking occurs, there is a

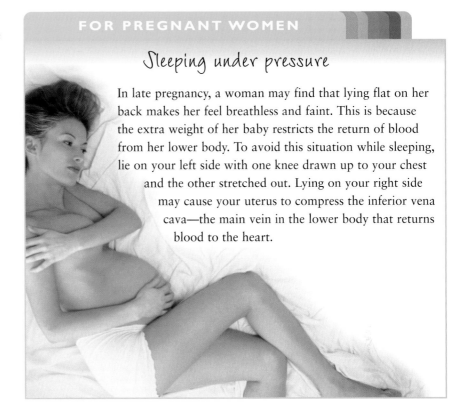

FOR PREGNANT WOMEN

Sleeping under pressure

In late pregnancy, a woman may find that lying flat on her back makes her feel breathless and faint. This is because the extra weight of her baby restricts the return of blood from her lower body. To avoid this situation while sleeping, lie on your left side with one knee drawn up to your chest and the other stretched out. Lying on your right side may cause your uterus to compress the inferior vena cava—the main vein in the lower body that returns blood to the heart.

sudden rise in heart rate and blood pressure, accompanied by a release of epinephrine. Some doctors have implicated this disruption to the normal low blood pressure during sleep in the development of high blood pressure. Some studies have shown that successful treatment of OSA, in some cases, can lead to a reduction in blood pressure.

SAFE SLEEPING FOR HEART PATIENTS

Most of us have a preferred sleeping position that we assume when we prepare for sleep, though during the night we may change position many times. For some people, however,

Heart attack patients have an increased need for sleep, often up to 12 hours a night.

certain positions, especially lying flat on the back, can exacerbate particular heart conditions.

People with poor heart function should avoid sleeping flat on their backs, which can bring on the symptoms of heart failure. The position causes an increase in the return of blood to the heart, raising its internal filling pressures. Sufferers can find themselves awakened by breathlessness, which can be relieved by sitting upright for several minutes.

If you have a heart condition and you want to avoid getting up in the middle of the night, try propping yourself up on a few pillows.

Rest for recovery

Rest is especially important when recovering from heart attack or heart failure. Hospitals may enforce an afternoon rest period and restrict visiting times so that patients can get the rest and sleep they need.

Sensible drinking

Do teetotalers have the right idea when it comes to alcohol and heart health? Or can a drink really be good for your heart? Read on for some surprising facts about alcohol and your cardiovascular system.

Alcohol hits your bloodstream just minutes after you have swallowed a drink (a little longer if you have lined your stomach with food). It has a range of effects on your blood, the blood vessels, and your heart itself. What are these effects and does it matter how much you drink?

A LITTLE OF WHAT YOU LIKE

Media reporting on the link between alcohol and cardiovascular health often leaves the heart-conscious public confused about whether or not to imbibe. In fact, the consensus seems to be to drink moderate amounts of alcohol on a regular basis.

Studies that have looked at alcohol consumption and the risk of heart disease find that moderate drinkers have a lower risk of heart disease than either teetotallers or heavy drinkers. Drinking within the guidelines for safe alcohol consumption is good for your heart in a number of ways.

Boosting good cholesterol

Moderate consumption of alcohol increases the blood concentration of good cholesterol—high-density lipoprotein (HDL). HDL is responsible for carrying excess cholesterol away from the artery walls and transporting it to the liver where it can be metabolized. In addition, alcohol seems to reduce levels of bad cholesterol—low-density lipoprotein (LDL). High levels of LDL are significant contributors to the development of atherosclerosis (clogging up of the blood vessels). The biggest benefits of moderate alcohol consumption are seen in men over 40 who have high levels of LDL cholesterol in their blood.

Free-flowing blood

In moderation, alcohol also has a beneficial effect on platelet function and the clotting system, including reducing fibrinogen—one of the proteins that causes blood to clot. It is these effects that are thought to cause the apparent protection from heart attack and stroke.

Add some fizz
Use mixers to keep your alcohol intake low. Try a refreshing spritzer—white wine mixed with sparkling mineral water—rather than a glass of wine alone.

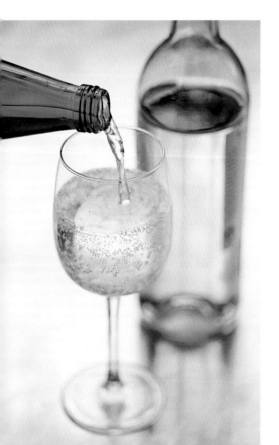

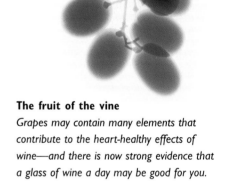

The fruit of the vine
Grapes may contain many elements that contribute to the heart-healthy effects of wine—and there is now strong evidence that a glass of wine a day may be good for you.

THE WINE STORY

Although the weight of evidence suggests that most of the beneficial effects of drinking relate to the alcohol itself, all alcoholic drinks contain many ingredients other than alcohol. Research carried out on wine, for example, has found evidence of antioxidants—chemicals that help to protect the body from free radicals. Free radicals are molecules that occur naturally in the body and are also produced by smoking, pollution, and sunlight. These molecules damage the arteries and can cause heart disease.

Red wine in particular is also thought to contain polyphenols,

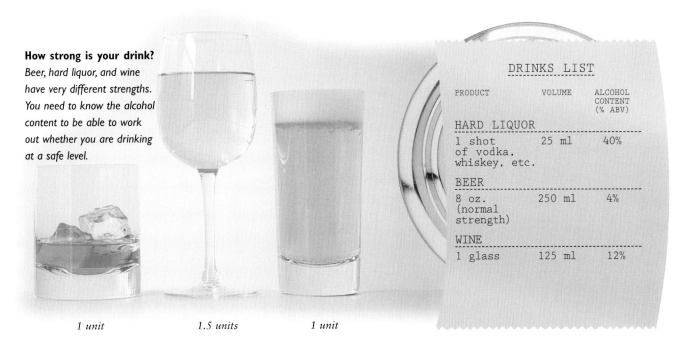

How strong is your drink?
Beer, hard liquor, and wine have very different strengths. You need to know the alcohol content to be able to work out whether you are drinking at a safe level.

DRINKS LIST		
PRODUCT	VOLUME	ALCOHOL CONTENT (% ABV)
HARD LIQUOR		
1 shot of vodka, whiskey, etc.	25 ml	40%
BEER		
8 oz. (normal strength)	250 ml	4%
WINE		
1 glass	125 ml	12%

1 unit   *1.5 units*   *1 unit*

which can inhibit clotting of the blood and widen constricted (narrowed) coronary arteries. Arterial relaxing and antiplatelet actions have also been observed, but their effects on cardiovascular health have not been fully studied.

Wine versus the rest

So, should we all be drinking wine instead of beer or hard liquor? Not necessarily. Some research into the health benefits of wine, compared with other alcoholic drinks, points to interesting variables. In the United States, wine drinkers tend to come from affluent backgrounds and have healthier lifestyles than beer and hard liquor drinkers. Studies over a period of six years, covering a combined sample of more than 300,000 people, have failed to show any significant advantage of one form of alcoholic drink over another when such variables are taken into account.

A SENSIBLE APPROACH

How can you be sure that you are drinking enough alcohol to bring out its cardiovascular benefits, but

not so much that the pleasure turns to pain?

The heart benefits of moderate alcohol consumption do not constitute an instruction to teetotallers to crack open a bottle of wine, nor do they invite occasional drinkers to step up their intake. These benefits do, however, reassure people who drink alcohol in moderation and warn them to keep an eye on their daily intake.

Know your units

The unit system used in the United Kingdom is designed to show how drinks compare and how much people are drinking in total. You can work out the number of units of alcohol in any drink by multiplying its volume (in liters) by its percentage of alcohol by volume. For example, a standard 75 cl bottle of wine with a 12 percent alcohol volume contains $0.75 \times 12 = 9$ units of alcohol.

Although many adults may have heard of measuring alcohol in units, few know the number of units in standard drinks such as wine and beer. There is now a move across Europe to label all alcoholic drinks in units, as well as volume and concentration, to help people gauge how much they are drinking.

The safe limits

Weighing the evidence, the British government has recommended a maximum of 3 to 4 units a day for men and 2 to 3 units for women. Guidelines by the U.S. government in *Nutrition and Health: Dietary Guidelines for Americans* recommend no more than 1 drink per day for women and 2 drinks for men. A U.S. standard "drink" contains 14 g of ethanol, however, whereas a British "drink" contains only 8 g.

Studies from more than 20 countries show that moderate drinkers have 20 to 40 percent less coronary heart disease than nondrinkers.

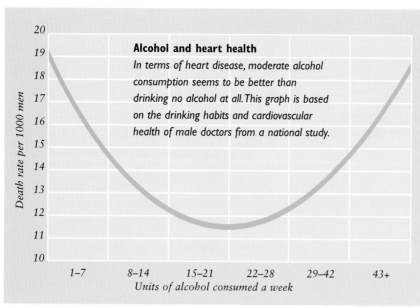

Alcohol and heart health
In terms of heart disease, moderate alcohol consumption seems to be better than drinking no alcohol at all. This graph is based on the drinking habits and cardiovascular health of male doctors from a national study.

Death rate per 1000 men: 10, 11, 12, 13, 14, 15, 16, 17, 18, 19, 20

Units of alcohol consumed a week: 1–7, 8–14, 15–21, 22–28, 29–42, 43+

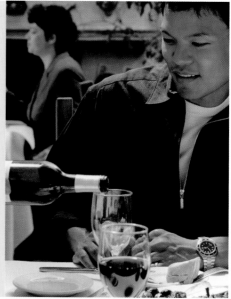

Alcohol on prescription?

TALKING POINT

Much of the evidence on the benefit of moderate drinking comes from questioning people on their drinking habits and then following up on them for a number of years. These studies show that people who drink moderate amounts of alcohol have fewer health problems than teetotalers or heavy drinkers. But factors other than alcohol may play a part. Moderate drinkers may eat a better diet or get more exercise, for example. Studies of alcohol-related problems such as cirrhosis of the liver find a direct link to the amount of alcohol consumed by society as a whole. So doctors don't prescribe drinking for teetotalers as a cardioprotective measure, but it's okay to continue drinking in moderation if you do so already.

AVOID BINGE DRINKING

Whatever your favored drink, it is clear that regular moderate drinking is much better for your heart than weekend binge drinking. Studies show that Scottish men derive no protective benefit from drinking, whereas Czech drinkers do. The difference is thought to be the result of drinking patterns. Men from the Czech Republic drink a moderate amount of beer each day, whereas the men involved in the Scottish study tended to follow a binge drinking pattern of consumption.

Binge drinking can also have more immediate health consequences: Palpitations can sometimes follow a night of overindulgence. The large injection of alcohol into the bloodstream stimulates the sympathetic nervous system and causes irregular heartbeat rhythms, also called arrhythmias. This condition is often referred to in Europe as "holiday heart," because of its association with weekend or holiday drinking. There is also some evidence to suggest that binge drinking can significantly raise blood pressure levels.

OVER THE LIMIT

Excessive alcohol consumption can directly damage your heart. It is the most commonly identified cause of heart muscle disease, resulting in heart enlargement and reduced function (dilated cardiomyopathy). Drinking heavily has been implicated in disturbances of heart rhythm, especially atrial fibrillation. There is also clear evidence that drinking more than 4 units of alcohol per day increases blood pressure.

Up to 10 percent of people with high blood pressure suffer the disease as a result of drinking more than 4 units of alcohol a day.

Drugs and the heart

Many illegal drugs can damage the cardiovascular system: In some cases the effects are fatal.

Cocaine

This drug stimulates the release of epinephrine and related hormones—the catecholamines—which have a prime impact upon the cardiovascular system. Cocaine also affects the heart's electrical activity by blocking sodium channels—the same property that is responsible for its local anesthetic effect. Heart rate and blood pressure rise within minutes of cocaine ingestion. This sudden rise in blood pressure can cause internal bleeding and stroke. In addition to speeding up the heart, it can have the opposite effect and slow the pulse rate to the point of death through a direct effect on the heart's conduction system. Cocaine can also cause spasm of the arteries, which can lead to a heart attack or stroke even in people with structurally normal coronary and cerebral arteries. This effect has been reported with any dosage and any route of ingestion. Long-term cocaine use has also been shown to accelerate atherosclerosis—clogging of the arteries—and can cause fibrosis and consequent heart failure.

Amphetamines

Like cocaine, amphetamines—also known as speed or uppers—cause the release of epinephrine, resulting in a rise in heart rate and blood pressure. Ecstasy is a related drug and its effects are similarly hazardous to the cardiovascular system. At the high doses often taken recreationally, amphetamines can cause palpitations and severe chest pain. Regular users also risk heart failure and damage to their blood vessels.

Opiates—morphine and heroin

Drugs such as morphine and heroine (diamorphine) are used in the medical treatment of acute (and occasionally chronic) heart pain and as part of the treatment of heart failure. They are effective because they dilate blood vessels, reduce breathlessness, and relieve anxiety. When they are taken in uncontrolled doses, however, they can lead to coma and, in rare cases, death from respiratory arrest.

Cannabis (Marijuana)

Contradictory effects of cannabis on the cardiovascular system have been reported, which may be due to differences in dosage. In young adults, 10 milligrams of cannabis causes a rise in heart rate of up to 90 beats per minute for approximately 1 hour. The drug also causes the major arteries to relax so that, although the amount of blood pumped by the heart increases by about 30 percent, there is only a small rise in blood pressure. But when the user stands up, the blood vessels cannot constrict, so blood may pool in the legs, instead of flowing up to the head, causing the person to faint. Large doses of cannabis can cause salt retention, with a more prolonged increase in blood volume, body weight, and blood pressure. Smoking cannabis reduces the oxygen-carrying capacity of the blood.

LSD

As well as being a hallucinogen, LSD causes an increase in heart rate and blood pressure. Blood pressure can rise by a small extent even with low doses.

Inhalants

A vast variety of compounds containing volatile solvents are abused. Acute intoxication can be very dangerous, causing arrhythmias brought on by the release of epinephrine. Long-term glue sniffing also has direct toxic effects on the heart.

Anabolic-androgenic steroids

Steroids have been used by some athletes and bodybuilders for many years. The drugs harm the cardiovascular system by increasing blood pressure. They can raise LDL cholesterol by up to 35 percent and lower HDL cholesterol by 60 percent. Steroids also increase platelet activity and blood thickness, further increasing risk of blood clots forming in the vessels. These changes increase the risk of heart attack and stroke.

Smoking—poisoning the heart

Most people associate smoking with lung disease, but in fact smoking is just as harmful for the heart as it is for the lungs. Tobacco smoke acts upon the cardiovascular system in a number of ways, all of which are damaging.

Smoking tobacco is the most important avoidable cause of chronic illness and early death in the developed world, causing a quarter of all deaths in middle-aged people. Smoking's role in lung cancer was proven first, but it is cardiovascular disease that is responsible for most smoking-related premature deaths.

THE NICOTINE ACTION

If you smoke, as you draw on a cigarette, the burning tobacco leaves transfer nicotine onto tiny droplets of tar, which are inhaled into your lungs. The drug is rapidly absorbed into the bloodstream and has many powerful effects on the nervous system—small doses of nicotine act as stimulants whereas large doses cause nerve paralysis.

Nicotine acts on the adrenal glands and nerve endings, causing the release of the hormones epinephrine and norepinephrine. Epinephrine increases heart rate and the heart's ability to contract; norepinephrine acts mainly to narrow the arteries. These two actions increase blood pressure, heart rate, and the amount of blood pumping through the heart by up to 20 percent.

The raised levels of epinephrine and norepinephrine in smokers increase the risk of disturbing the heart's rhythm, resulting in arrhythmias. This can be simply a nuisance with occasional palpitations or an irregularity of the heart beat that reduces the heart's pumping efficiency. In some cases, however, arrhythmias are life threatening, with complete collapse of the circulation. Arrhythmias are the most common cause of sudden death in people with coronary artery disease.

HEART-BREAKING HABIT

Smoking damages the cardiovascular system. It causes angina (chest pain), heart attacks, peripheral vascular disease, aortic aneurysm, and stroke. Smoking is thought to exert its harmful effects in three main ways.

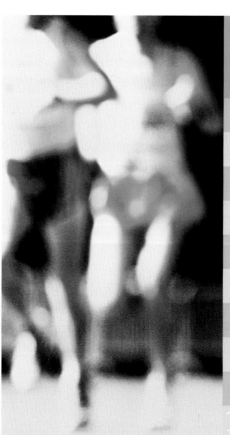

10 Great reasons to stop smoking

You don't have to look hard to find evidence of the damaging effects of smoking on the cardiovascular system. Use this list to motivate you to quit.

1 Smoking doubles your risk of dying of coronary artery disease.

2 Smoking causes ischemia—lack of oxygen in the bloodstream caused by the clogging of arteries. This condition increases the risk of a heart attack by 70 percent.

3 The death rate from dilation and rupture of the aorta (aortic aneurysm) in smokers is at least six times that in people who do not smoke.

4 Most people with narrowing of the leg arteries—peripheral vascular disease— serious enough to limit their walking smoked at some point in their lives.

5 Only 59 percent of 35-year-old women who smoke will still be alive at 75. In contrast, 75 percent of nonsmokers will live to at least 75.

6 Only 41 percent of 35-year-old men who smoke will still be alive at 75. This figure compares with 65 percent in nonsmokers.

7 Smokers who are in their 30s and 40s have at least five times as many heart attacks as nonsmokers of these ages.

8 Each cigarette shortens a smoker's lifespan by about 5 minutes.

9 About 20 percent of all deaths are attributable to smoking—more than all fatalities caused by road accidents, alcohol, murder, suicide, AIDS, illegal drugs, and fire.

10 Every hour in the United States, 45 people die of a smoking-related illness.

Accelerating atherosclerosis

Smoking causes a build-up of plaque in the walls of arteries. Cholesterol is the raw material of fatty plaque, but it is damage to the delicate endothelium lining in all blood vessels that allows deposition of cholesterol and other molecules and cells. This sets up an inflammatory process that results in the formation of clogging plaque. By damaging the endothelium, smoking causes the endothelial cells to swell. As plaques grow and change shape, their surface is in a state of flux and can rupture, thereby exposing collagen along with other molecules that activate the body's clotting system. This is thought to trigger most heart attacks and strokes.

Provoking thrombosis

In order to live, our bodies must constantly balance the formation and breakdown of blood clots. Clotting is essential to life—Without it we would bleed to death after a minor cut or bruise. But if clotting continued unchecked, the blood would turn to jelly and stop flowing altogether. Smoking alters this delicate balance, tilting it toward the possibility of a clot blocking a blood vessel—thrombosis.

Blood clots are made up of tiny blood cells (platelets) linked together by chains of fibrin—a stringy protein—and other molecules. Smoking increases platelet binding and adherence to the endothelium, partly by increasing the concentration of fatty acids in the blood. It also increases the formation of fibrinogen, which forms fibrin.

Smoking while on the oral contraceptive pill can increase the risk of thrombosis further.

Inhibiting thrombolysis

The body naturally breaks down potential clots in the bloodstream by a process called thrombolysis. But smoking gets in the way of this process by reducing the activity of the body's own "clot-buster"—tissue plasminogen activator.

PASSIVE SMOKING RISKS

When you breathe in the same air as a cigarette smoker, not only are you inhaling the cigarette smoke, but you are also taking in the smoker's exhaled breath—which contains smoke particles and gases. Just like first-hand smoking, passive smoking increases your heart rate, blood pressure and blood levels of car-bon monoxide. It also decreases the blood's oxygen-carrying capacity and HDL (good) cholesterol, increasing platelet binding and damaging the lining of blood vessels.

A real danger

There is new evidence that passive smoking can increase your risk of coronary artery disease by 25 percent. This is less than that estimated for active smoking (70 percent) but, as nearly half of adults and children are exposed to passive smoke in their own homes or public places,

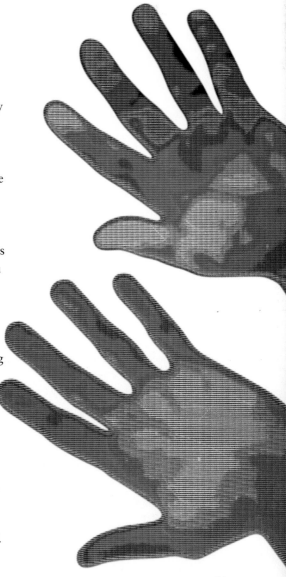

Cold smoke
Smokers can suffer from cold hands due to a reduction in blood flow to the hands (top right). One of the reasons for this is that components of tobacco smoke cause the arteries in these areas to become narrowed.

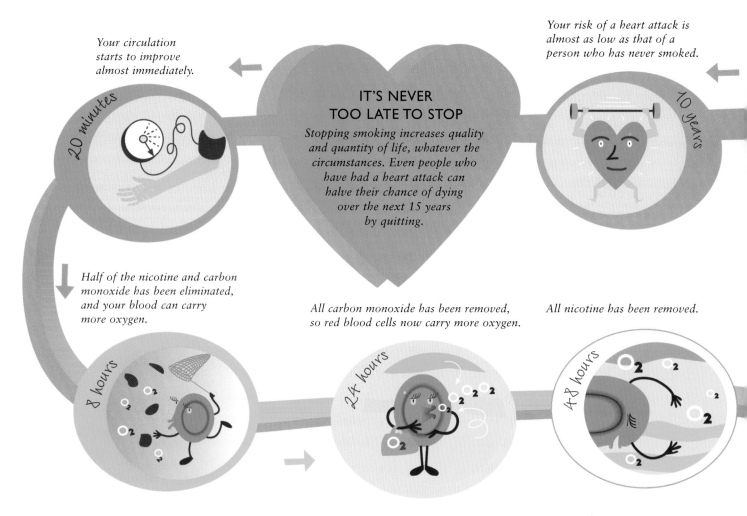

Your circulation starts to improve almost immediately.

20 minutes

Your risk of a heart attack is almost as low as that of a person who has never smoked.

10 years

IT'S NEVER TOO LATE TO STOP

Stopping smoking increases quality and quantity of life, whatever the circumstances. Even people who have had a heart attack can halve their chance of dying over the next 15 years by quitting.

Half of the nicotine and carbon monoxide has been eliminated, and your blood can carry more oxygen.

All carbon monoxide has been removed, so red blood cells now carry more oxygen.

All nicotine has been removed.

8 hours

24 hours

48 hours

---

this represents a major public health problem. One study (1992) reported that children of parents who smoke inhale the equivalent of 60 to 150 cigarettes a year.

PATTERNS OF SMOKING

More than 75 million people in the United States smoke. Smokers in the general population are fewer since 1965 (45.5 percent vs. 26.8 percent in 2000), but the U.S. government wants a more marked decrease by 2010 (12 percent). In recent years, these numbers have see-sawed (22.9 percent in 1991; 26.4 in 1992; 28.7 in 1997). In general, the following can be said about U.S. smokers:

• More men than women smoke, (28.5 vs. 25.1), but more women than men are starting.

• Among racial/ethnic groups, Hispanics (18.1 percent) and Asians/Pacific Islanders (15.1 percent) had the lowest prevalence, whereas American Indians and Alaska Natives had the highest (40.8 percent).

• Those earning a General Equivalency Diploma (GED) had the highest prevalence (44.4 percent) compared with people with masters, professional, and doctoral degrees (8.5 percent).

• Adults living below the poverty level had the highest smoking prevalence by socio-economic group (33.3 percent).

• Of high school students, 28.5 percent currently smoke, down from 36.4 percent in 1997 and 34.8 percent in 1999.

THE HEALTHY OPTION

More than 70 percent of smokers in the United States today have made at least one attempt to quit, and approximately 46 percent try to quit each year. Most smokers make several attempts before they are successful.

STUB OUT THE HABIT

Everyone has a slightly different way of quitting smoking, and you have to find the strategy that is right for you. There are, however, tactics that many people have found useful, ones that can increase your chances of long-term success.

Set a date

Many people find it helpful to make an occasion of quitting by choosing a memorable day—no-smoking day, an

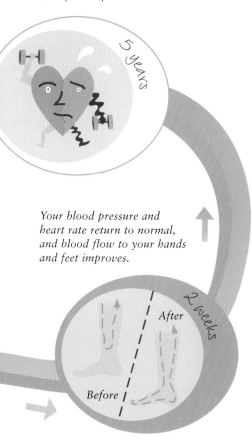

Your risk of a heart attack is half that of a smoker.

5 years

Your blood pressure and heart rate return to normal, and blood flow to your hands and feet improves.

2 weeks

After

Before

Nonsmokers have a more than 70 percent increase in risk of stroke if they live with a smoker.

anniversary, birthday, or, as tradition often dictates, the first day of the year.

Tell the world

Talk to your doctor, dentist, family, and friends about your reasons for quitting and how you are planning to do it. Their support will be invaluable in the days, weeks, and months ahead.

Paradoxically, some people find it better to follow the opposite of this strategy and tell no one. Find the way that works for you.

Use nicotine substitutes

Many people find nicotine replacement helpful, and research suggests that it should double your chances of success. The replacements come in many different forms, including

chewing gum, inhalers, sublingual (under the tongue) tablets, or even nasal sprays. Treatment with nicotine replacement aims to ease you off nicotine over a three-month period. Clear instructions are provided in the packages. For example, 15-mg patches are used daily for eight weeks, followed by 10-mg patches for two weeks and then 5-mg patches for another two weeks.

Because all these preparations contain nicotine, it is sensible to discuss nicotine replacement therapy with your doctor before quitting, but in most cases it is safer than the alternative of carrying on smoking.

Avoid temptation

Throw away all your cigarettes, lighters, and ashtrays; make your house a smoke-free zone. Plan what to do in the situations where you used to smoke; in the early days it may be safer to avoid places where you smoked or bought cigarettes.

Count your pennies

A satisfying, and distracting, exercise is to work out exactly how much money you will save per day, week, month, year, and the rest of your life. Use the money to save up for something you would not otherwise have.

Coping with withdrawal

Remember that it is normal to experience withdrawal symptoms and cravings—it's simply your body's way of recovering from years of smoking. Try taking deep breaths or going for a short walk, but avoid eating sweets,

as this is the main reason for weight gain immediately after quitting— Instead, eat pieces of fruit, drink water, or chew sugar-free gum.

Keep on trying

If you don't succeed the first time, keep trying. Most smokers make several attempts before they stamp out the habit forever. But did you know that more than 3,000 people in the United States quit for good every day?

Remember, there is always help available from family and friends or by contacting QuitNet (see page 160).

Spend, spend, spend
Treat yourself to some of life's little luxuries with the money you save by not smoking. It's not just the pennies that count, though; your heart and circulatory system will be much better off with a smoke-free you.

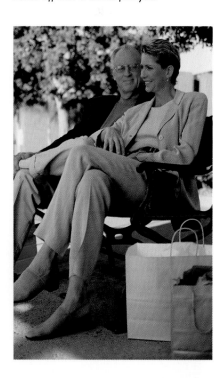

The caffeine conundrum

A cup of coffee can provide a kick-start in the morning and a welcome pick-me-up throughout the day, but too much could give you palpitations. Find out more about caffeine's complex effects on the cardiovascular system.

Over the first hour after a single cup of coffee, heart rate falls.

The concentration of caffeine in the blood peaks between 15 minutes and 2 hours after drinking coffee, depending on the individual.

By 3 hours, the heart rate rises above baseline. The effects take between 5 and 6 hours to wear off. In pregnant women and newborns, however, the effects can last up to 100 hours.

Caffeine has a tachyphylactic effect — you need to drink more and more to get the same buzz.

Coffee is a highly complex mixture of water, proteins, organic acids, minerals, sugars, caffeine, and fats. An 8-ounce cup of roasted, ground coffee can contain between 95 and 280 milligrams of caffeine, whereas a cup of instant coffee contains 65 to 280 milligrams. Coffee is not the only food that contains caffeine—it is also found in tea, chocolate and some soft drinks.

ACTING ON THE HEART

Caffeine affects the cardiovascular system in three ways:

- It blocks the body's receptors for adenosine. Adenosine has a direct effect on the heart's electrical conduction system—A few milligrams injected intravenously can stop the heart beating.
- It blocks some of the actions of phosphodiesterases, enzymes involved in the chain of effects triggered by epinephrine.
- It causes the release of calcium from the intracellular stores.

These three actions, all of which vary according to dose, interact and underlie caffeine's complex cardiovascular effects.

MODERATION IS KEY

At face value, caffeine seems to have alarming effects on the cardiovascular system. It causes concentrations of both epinephrine and norepinephrine to increase significantly, raising cardiac output and blood pressure. It also causes some blood vessels in the body to constrict and some to enlarge. This action, coupled with an increase in blood platelet binding, could be a recipe for disaster in terms of risk of clotting. Some studies also suggest that heavy coffee consumption—six cups a day for six weeks—increases levels of LDL (bad) cholesterol, whereas levels of HDL (good) cholesterol fall. When caffeine is sensibly consumed, however, these potential problems cannot reach fruition—Consumed in moderation, caffeine is not dangerous in terms of cardiovascular health. Susceptible individuals, such as people with cardiac arrhythmias, are advised to watch their intake.

Dutch scientists found a 9 to 14 percent rise in blood levels of cholesterol after drinking pressed (cafetière) coffee; filtered coffee had no effect.

MORE THAN JUST A BUZZ

"Caffeinism"—the excessive consumption of caffeine—causes a variety of nervous and physical effects, including a feeling of anxiety, disturbance of sleep and mood swings. It occurs usually when consumption exceeds 500 milligrams a day—the equivalent of about three strong cups of filtered coffee. By drinking excessive amounts of coffee on a regular basis, your heart may start to suffer and you could begin to experience palpitations.

If you think you are taking in too much caffeine, you should try to reduce your consumption. Try to limit your intake of caffeine-containing drinks to one or two per day.

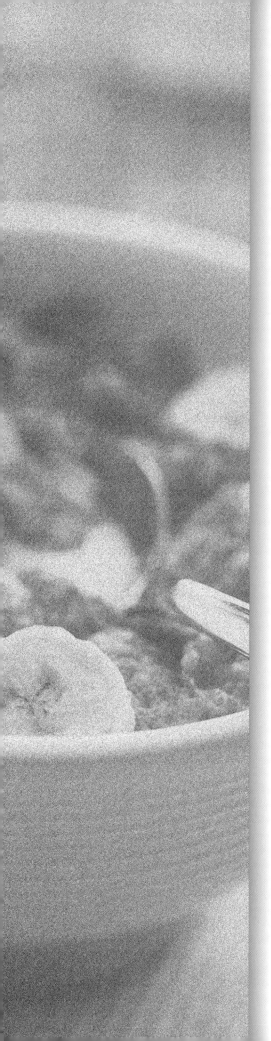

EAT A HEART-HEALTHY DIET

Food choices have far-reaching implications for your cardiovascular health. Too much fat in the diet is a major culprit in coronary artery disease—arteries become clogged up and more easily blocked. Eating a varied, balanced diet, low in saturated fat and high in fiber and fresh produce can pay dividends on the heart health front. In addition to providing cardioprotective antioxidant vitamins, fruit and vegetables play an important part in maintaining a healthy weight—another factor crucial to a healthy heart.

 66   *Tip the scales in favor of a heart-healthy diet. Make the switch to less fat and more healthy fruit and vegetables.*

 73   *Learn about the superfoods that can help to keep your heart and blood vessels in peak condition.*

 76   *Is your weight putting a strain on your heart? Find out what's a healthy weight and motivate yourself to lose any excess baggage.*

Food for your heart

Eating for a healthy heart needn't be hard work—It's a question of balance. Make simple food changes to tip the scales in favor of a low-fat, high-fiber diet, and your heart and circulation will reap the benefits.

On the next few pages we explain how the main food components influence heart health. Read on to find out if your diet could offer your heart more protection.

FAT—FRIEND OR FOE?

For the health or diet-conscious, "fat" is a dirty word—it clogs up arteries, piles on the pounds, and puts the heart under pressure. But fat is also a concentrated source of energy that provides us with vital calories. It is an important source of essential fatty acids, it aids the delivery of fat-soluble vitamins (A, D, E, and K), and it helps to protect internal organs and keep us warm. Health problems stem from eating too much fat and from eating the wrong type, because not all fats are the same.

Types of fat

Fats can be divided into two basic types: saturated and unsaturated. The latter encompasses both mono-unsaturated and polyunsaturated fats. All fats are built from the same building blocks—carbon, hydrogen, and oxygen. Carbon atoms form the backbone of each fat molecule and are linked together in chains of varying length and shape. Hydrogen atoms attach to each carbon atom. Whether or not a fat is saturated depends on whether each carbon atom has a full complement of hydrogen atoms attached. If it has, then the fat molecule is said to be "saturated" with hydrogen. The degree of saturation determines if a fat is solid or liquid: The more saturated it is, the more solid it is. Saturated fats are found mainly in meat and dairy products, although coconut also has a very high saturated fat content.

Bad fat

Excessive intake of saturated fats and trans fats has been clearly linked to coronary artery disease. Trans fats are made when vegetable oils are packed with extra hydrogen (hydrogenated) to make them solid for use in processed foods such as cookies and for certain margarines. (Not all margarines contain trans

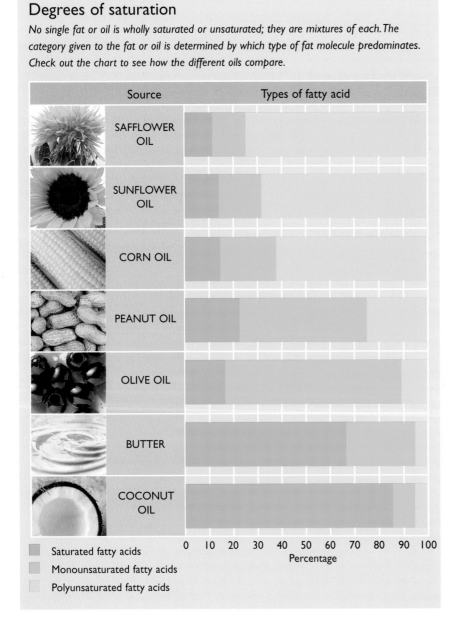

Degrees of saturation

No single fat or oil is wholly saturated or unsaturated; they are mixtures of each. The category given to the fat or oil is determined by which type of fat molecule predominates. Check out the chart to see how the different oils compare.

Source	Types of fatty acid
SAFFLOWER OIL	
SUNFLOWER OIL	
CORN OIL	
PEANUT OIL	
OLIVE OIL	
BUTTER	
COCONUT OIL	

0 10 20 30 40 50 60 70 80 90 100
Percentage

■ Saturated fatty acids
■ Monounsaturated fatty acids
■ Polyunsaturated fatty acids

FATWISE IS HEARTWISE

How can you put your knowledge of good fat and bad fat into practice? Here are some practical tips for tailoring your fat consumption for a healthy heart by choosing and cooking your food wisely.

IN THE SUPERMARKET

- *Choose lean cuts of meat or go for chicken and fish instead.*
- *Choose skim or low-fat milk, reduced-fat cheeses and low-fat yogurt.*
- *Avoid processed foods that contain palm oil, coconut oil, and cocoa butter.*
- *Choose low-fat snacks, such as pretzels and dried fruit, instead of chips, chocolate, and cookies.*
- *Choose low-fat spreads and unsaturated margarines that are virtually free from trans (hydrogenated) fats.*

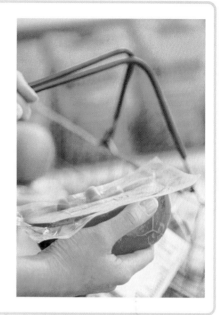

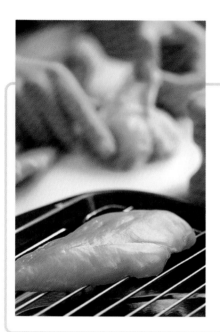

IN THE KITCHEN

- *Always remove the skin from poultry and trim off any visible fat from meat before cooking.*
- *Grill, steam, poach, microwave, stir-fry, boil, or bake rather than frying or deep frying.*
- *Avoid adding or cooking in unnecessary fat—For example, dry roast poultry and cuts of meat on a rack over the roasting pan to allow fat to drain off.*

- *Before making gravy, skim off all the fat from the meat juices.*
- *Use unsaturated cooking oil. Mono-unsaturated fats are preferable to polyunsaturated fats because they are stable at high temperatures.*
- *Occasionally replace meat with oily fish, beans, or lentils.*

IN THE RESTAURANT

- *Avoid high-fat appetizers such as pâté or anything deep fried—opt for melon, soup, or smoked salmon.*
- *When you order, don't be afraid to tell the waiter that you would like your vegetables served without butter or your fish without sauce.*
- *Avoid creamy sauces, pastry, and anything fried.*

- *Vegetarian options are not always lower in saturated fat—avoid dishes containing a lot of cheese.*
- *You don't have to miss out on dessert— Just choose wisely. Fruit-based puddings, sorbets, and meringues are delicious, heart-healthy choices.*

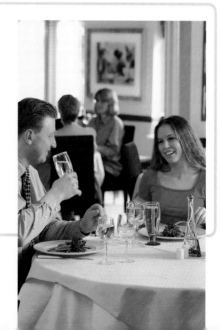

fats—Some major brands of sunflower and olive oil margarines use a different process.)

Research shows that saturated fats and trans fats increase both total cholesterol levels in the blood and levels of the harmful low-density lipoprotein (LDL) cholesterol. For this reason, it is important to reduce the level of saturated and trans fats in the diet, replacing these with poly-unsaturates and monounsaturates.

Good fat

In contrast, unsaturated fats, found mainly in vegetable foods, can help to lower LDL cholesterol levels, particularly when they replace saturated fat in the diet. Poly-unsaturated fats are found in vegetable oils, nuts, and seeds, while monounsaturated fatty acids are found in some nuts as well as in olive, groundnut, and rapeseed oils. A subgroup of polyunsaturated fats, known as the omega essential fatty acids, are of particular importance to cardiovascular health. Omega-3 fatty acids (which come mainly from oily fish such as mackerel, sardines, and salmon, and also from rapeseed oil) make blood less sticky and so less likely to clot and cause heart disease.

Most of the cholesterol in the blood is made by the liver from foods rich in saturated fat—only about 25 percent comes from foods high in cholesterol.

Moderate your fat intake

To benefit your cardiovascular system, you don't need to cut fat out of your diet entirely; the main change you need to make is in the type of fat you eat—less saturated, more unsaturated. No more than 33 percent of your total energy intake should come from fat of any sort, and no more than a third of that should come from saturated fat.

On a practical level, for an average woman eating 1920 kilocalories a day. this translates into a maximum daily intake of 70 grams fat, of which no more than 23 grams should be saturated fat. For an average man eating 2550 kilocalories a day, the figures are 90 grams fat in total and 30 grams saturated fat.

Be a "fat" detective

Information labels on food identify the types of fat they contain. Try to get into the habit of inspecting these labels; you'll be surprised by how the grams of fat add up, even in so-called "95 percent fat-free" foods.

Experts recommend that we should increase our intake of foods that are rich in omega-3 fatty acids, since the average Western diet is typically low in these cardioprotective nutrients. You can easily pack in a couple of servings a week—for example by eating grilled salmon for a weekend breakfast or using a little tuna salad for a delicious baked potato filling. If you are not a great fan of oily fish, you could take a daily fish oil supplement and also look out for foods fortified with fish oil, or eat eggs from chickens fed omega-3 fatty acids.

Keep an eye on cholesterol

The key to low cholesterol levels is reducing your intake of saturated fat; but what about high-cholesterol foods such as eggs? Should you be cutting down on these foods, too? Although eggs and shellfish, such as shrimp, are reasonably high in cholesterol, they are low in saturated fat; it's fine to enjoy these foods within a balanced low-fat diet.

High levels of LDL cholesterol can cause clogging of arteries—atherosclerosis—and contribute to the risk of heart disease. Keep your cholesterol levels under control by choosing heart-healthy foods.

CARDIAC CARBOHYDRATES

The carbohydrate banner includes fiber, starches (complex carbo-hydrates) and sugars (simple carbohydrates). Each type affects your heart and circulation differently.

How do cholesterol-lowering margarines work and who should be using them?

Cholesterol-reducing spreads contain plant stanol esters, which helps to block absorption of cholesterol. Studies have found that these spreads can reduce total and "bad" LDL cholesterol by 10 to 15 percent, and so they may be useful diet aids for those concerned about cholesterol. People taking lipid-lowering drugs should use them as a supplement, but not a replacement, for drug therapy. Pregnant women should use them only after consultation with a doctor.

ASK THE EXPERT

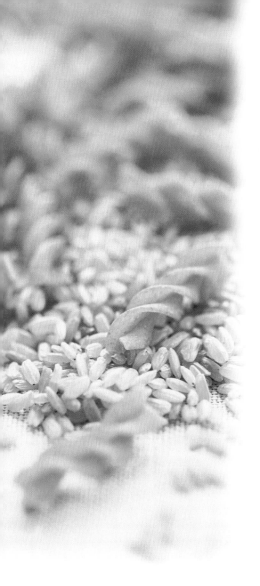

Choose the high-fiber alternative
Brown rice and whole wheat pasta have more fiber than white varieties. By choosing foods that are high in fiber you can help to reduce the level of cholesterol in your blood.

Cholesterol-lowering fiber

Also known as nonstarch polysaccharide (NSP), dietary fiber comes in two forms—water insoluble and water soluble.

- **Insoluble fiber** This type of fiber is found in wholegrain starchy foods, such as bread, pasta, breakfast cereals, brown rice, and bran. Increasing your intake of insoluble fiber can help to reduce the risk of heart disease, and the protective effect seems most closely linked with long-term cereal fiber intake. Cereal lowers LDL cholesterol levels in the blood, possibly by decreasing the amount of fat that is actually absorbed by the stomach.

- **Water-soluble fiber** Found in peas, beans, oats, barley, nuts, seeds, fruit, and vegetables. Soluble fiber can contribute to cholesterol reduction when included in a diet that is already low in saturated fat. It does this through a variety of mechanisms, one of which is through binding to cholesterol in the stomach and preventing its absorption.

High fiber equals more fluids

Fiber consumption increases the body's need for fluids because it absorbs water as food travels through the digestive tract. A healthy water intake is normally about eight glasses a day; if you're boosting your fiber intake, then step up your water intake too—About 10 to 12 glasses should help to compensate for the extra fiber and prevent constipation.

Maximize starch intake

A heart-healthy diet is based on complex carbohydrate; ensure that at least half of your daily calories are provided by a mixture of fiber-rich foods. Swinging the balance toward starchy foods, such as bread, potatoes, whole-grain cereals, pasta, legumes, fruit, and vegetables, is central to a high-fiber, low-fat diet.

You may already be eating heart-friendly meals without knowing it: Pasta with a tomato-based sauce and a green salad is a quick and easy-to-prepare evening meal that is low in fat and high in fiber. Other great cardioprotective meals include a hearty bean casserole, smoked salmon, and scrambled eggs; even a baked potato with low-fat cheddar cheese scores high on the heart health scale.

positive health tips

Easy ways to lower LDL cholesterol

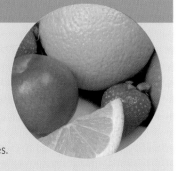

- Eat plenty of fruit and vegetables for their excellent supply of the antioxidant vitamins beta-carotene and C, both of which help prevent LDL cholesterol from becoming oxidized and deposited in your heart's arteries.

- Increase your intake of water-soluble fiber, which is found in legumes, oats, nuts, and apples, as it can help to lower high blood cholesterol levels.

- Keep your intake of saturated fats to a minimum. Foods rich in saturated fat encourage the liver to manufacture LDL cholesterol.

- Keep your intake of trans fats to an absolute minimum. Most margarines now include trans fat percentages on their labels, so you can make a healthy choice, but some are hidden within cookies, cakes, and dairy products.

Mix and match

By building up a repertoire of healthy breakfasts, lunches, and dinners, you can then mix and match them to create varied daily menus that will never be boring.

Minimize sugar consumption

High-sugar foods are effectively nutritionally "empty," in that they provide no other benefit except calories. While there is no evidence that sugar promotes coronary artery disease directly, overeating sugary foods increases the likelihood of being overweight—a risk factor for heart problems—and may increase levels in the blood of a fat called triglyceride (see page 42). Do the following to avoid excess intake of sugar:

- Double-check food packaging for hidden ingredients—Sucrose, glucose, dextrose, fructose, and maltose are all sugars.
- Cut down on sugar in hot drinks, and choose low-calorie, sugar-free, or unsweetened soft drinks.
- Opt for fresh fruit or unsweetened varieties of yogurt instead of chocolate and cakes.
- Avoid sugar-coated cereals. Some are not as obvious as others—Muesli can contain lots of hidden sugar, so check the label.
- Try halving the sugar in recipes.
- Use low-sugar varieties of ready-made puddings and desserts.

EAT THE BEST PROTEIN

Proteins are essential for growth and repair within the body, but in most developed countries, people eat too much protein. Excess protein is not beneficial—If not used as energy, the extra calories provided by this vital food component are stored as fat. Continuous overeating of protein-

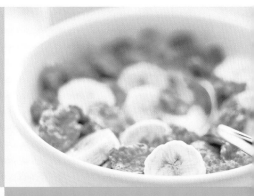

Breakfast

Folate fortified cereal with low-fat milk and a banana.

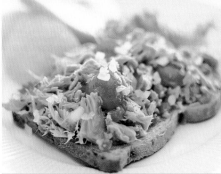

Lunch

Tuna on wholegrain bread with lettuce and tomato, and a pear.

Dinner

Small salmon fillet, yogurt-based sauce, large portion of spinach, sweetcorn, and green salad.

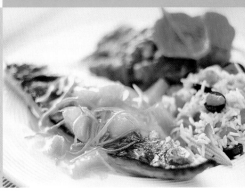

rich foods, such as meat, fish, and dairy products, can increase the risk of being overweight, which is closely linked to heart disease.

Animal or vegetable?

The type of protein you eat—whether it is plant or animal in origin—dictates how much saturated fat it contributes to your diet. Protein intake in the Western world is mainly from animal sources, such as meat, fish, eggs, cheese, and milk—All of which, except fish, are high in saturated fat. Most of us in developed countries get a smaller amount of protein from plant protein, such as legumes, cereals, and nuts, which are low in saturated fat. By changing the balance between

animal and plant sources of protein in your diet and increasing the latter, you can boost your heart health. One plant protein, soy, has been proven especially beneficial to cardiovascular health because it contains phytoestrogens (see page 74).

If you eat meat, you don't have to go completely vegetarian, but having a couple of meat-free days each week is a good start on the road to better heart health. Initially, you may find it easier to substitute fish—for example, a salmon steak instead of a lamb chop. When choosing milk, butter, cheese, and cream, opt for low-fat versions where possible and select lean cuts of meat. The amount of fat, particularly saturated fat, in your diet will be slashed.

Breakfast

Grapefruit segments and a slice of toast with low-fat, poly-unsaturated margarine and a little marmalade.

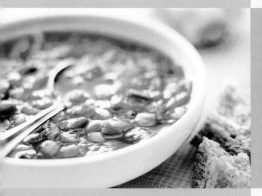

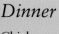

Lunch

Mixed bean soup with whole grain bread, followed by a fruit salad.

Dinner

Chicken casserole with onions and mushrooms, served with carrots and broccoli and a baked potato. Finish off with fresh fruit and low-fat yogurt.

MIRACLE MICRONUTRIENTS AND SUPPLEMENTS

As well as providing a mixture of protein, carbohydrate, and fat, foods also contain traces of other natural chemicals—enzymes, vitamins or minerals—that can benefit cardiovascular health. Sometimes it's worthwhile taking a supplement of a particular micronutrient to ensure you get the maximum cardiac benefit. Ask your doctor for advice before taking any supplements.

Heart-friendly antioxidants

Once it was purely a technical term, but antioxidant has become a real heart buzzword. Antioxidants are thought to help neutralize free radicals, harmful molecules in the body that promote atherosclerosis. It is clear that low intakes of antioxidants are associated with a high risk of heart disease; populations that consume large amounts of antioxidant-rich foods, such as the Greeks and Italians, have a low incidence of coronary artery disease.

The principal antioxidant nutrients are vitamins C and E and the carotenoids—particularly beta-carotene, which the body converts to vitamin A, and the lycopenes, responsible for the red color in tomatoes. Other antioxidants include selenium, manganese, zinc, and chemicals called flavonoids.

Sodium and potassium

One of the consequences of modern food processing has been not only to increase the sodium content of foods, but also to decrease potassium. Sodium and potassium work in partnership in the body, and the actions of each are balanced by the other. By ensuring that you eat enough foods rich in potassium, you can promote the removal of excess sodium, which can help to prevent high blood pressure. A potassium-packed banana is a tasty standby snack and is great for your circulation. See the next page for more on the link between sodium and your cardiovascular health.

The B vitamins

A high level of a chemical called homocysteine in blood is associated with atherosclerosis, making it a risk factor for heart disease. Folic acid (the synthetic version of the

Fill up on fantastic fish

Fish is an excellent protein provider that is also low in saturated fat and rich in omega-3 fatty acids (oily fish being the richest source). Studies show that eating just one oily fish meal a week can halve a person's risk of sudden cardiac death. Try to eat such meals once or twice a week—a grilled salmon steak or baked mackerel make a quick evening meal, or for lunch have a sardine sandwich or a smoked salmon bagel. Other fish high in omega-3 include trout, tuna, red mullet, and anchovies.

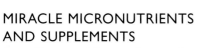

B vitamin folate) has been shown to lower levels of homocysteine in the bloodstream. Folate can be difficult for the body to absorb; therefore, in addition to eating naturally folate-rich foods (such as spinach, broccoli and oranges), it is worth increasing your intake of folic acid–fortified foods (such as breakfast cereal) and taking a daily supplement. Studies have shown that a 200-milligram folic acid supplement lowers homocysteine in healthy people by about 30 percent.

SALT CONTENT

PRODUCT	WEIGHT (g)	SALT CONTENT (mg)
CANNED FOODS		
Baked beans	100	500
Red kidney beans	100	390
Pasta sauce	100	470
Soup	100	400-800
CEREALS/BREAD		
Cornflakes	100	1100
Bread	100	500-550
CHIPS/SAVORY SNACKS		
Onion rings	100	1600
Potato chips	100	1600
SAUCES AND PICKLES		
Tomato ketchup	100	1160
Sandwich pickle	100	1302
COLD MEATS		
Cured ham	100	860
Pepperoni	100	1447

Co-enzyme Q10 (CoQ10)

Essential for the release of energy from food, this enzyme occurs in a range of foods and is also produced naturally within the body, although production may decline with age or during illness. Studies have shown that CoQ10 deficiencies exist in people with heart disease.

SALT OF THE EARTH

Small amounts of salt—sodium chloride—are essential in our diet, but most of us eat far more than we need. Many experts agree that a high salt intake is a major factor in the development of high blood pressure and that reducing sodium intake can reduce blood pressure. The current average intake is around 9 grams of salt a day, and latest guidelines suggest this should be cut to a daily maximum of 6 grams.

Full of flavor

You may think the easiest way to reduce the amount of salt you eat is to cut back on the amount you add when cooking or at the table—and, of course, this is an obvious starting point. But a surprising amount of salt is hidden within foods. The more

Check out sodium at the supermarket
Sodium, in its many forms, is often hidden within foods, especially processed and ready-made foods. As much as 75 percent of the salt in our diet comes from processed foods.

salt we eat, the more we seem to like it. If you gradually reduce the amount of salt you eat, your palate will adapt as the salt receptors on the tongue regain their natural sensitivity. The process of retraining the palate takes about four weeks, but you'll soon find you prefer foods with less salt. Try using herbs, spices, lemon, or mustard to pep up your food—you'll be surprised at how delicious low-sodium food can be.

- Begin using less salt in cooking and at the table; cut down gradually.
- Choose reduced-sodium foods when available.
- Cut down on salty snack foods such as peanuts and chips.
- Reduce your intake of highly salted processed foods, such as packaged and canned soups and sauces, and other prepackaged foods.

Know your labels

Salt is made up of the elements sodium and chloride, but it is only the sodium part that we need to keep an eye on. Other additives based on sodium that you should watch out for include monosodium glutamate (MSG, a flavor enhancer), sodium nitrate (a preservative), sodium bicarbonate (a leavening agent), and sodium saccharin (a sweetener).

The nutritional information on food labels usually gives a figure for the amount of sodium per 100 grams or per serving. As a general rule, if a food contains less than 0.1 gram (100 mg) sodium per serving, it is reasonably low in salt; if there is more than 0.5 gram (500 mg) per serving, it has too much.

Heart-healthy eating for life

When it comes to cardiovascular health, it seems that the Greeks and Italians take first place. What can we learn from these heart-healthy people and what can we do to encourage healthy eating habits throughout life?

Eating a healthy diet can help you to live longer and remain healthier; it can also protect you against heart disease. When it comes to heart-healthy eating, begin like you plan to continue—make simple changes for life. Starting as early as possible can have significant impact on your risk of heart problems in later life.

LAYING THE FOUNDATIONS FOR GOOD HEART HEALTH

Several studies show that nutrition in infancy and childhood can have implications on our health in later life. The development of the fatty streaks and atheroma—the first signs of heart disease—start in early childhood. During our children's formative years we should help them to lay down heart-healthy roots.

It's never too early to begin thinking about healthy eating. Babies and toddlers have high energy and nutrient requirements and small stomachs, and so warrant special consideration. A high-fiber, low-fat diet is not recommended for the under-fives because it does not supply all their nutritional needs. Once children are over the age of five, help to keep their fat intake low by switching to lower fat dairy products, such as low-fat milk and yogurts.

A happy balance
A balanced range of healthy foods is the key to a healthy heart. As part of a social occasion, meals are even better when unrushed and shared with family or friends.

Growing needs
Teenage years are a period of rapid growth, and they are often accompanied by what can seem like an insatiable appetite. Encourage teenagers to fill up on fruit and vegetables and energy-dense starchy foods such as whole-grain bread, pasta, rice, and unsweetened breakfast cereals.

Vegetarian diets
People often worry that a vegetarian diet won't provide all the essential nutrients needed for all-around health, including that of the heart and circulation. In recent years the number of vegeterians in the United States has increased; today, as many as 20 percent of the population purchase vegeterian products, and about 1 percent consider themselves strict vegeterians (never eat animal

Filling the gaps in your diet

Research suggests that cardiac protection begins in the uterus and eating well throughout pregnancy is essential to ensure your baby has a healthy heart. Recent studies have linked babies with high birthweights to a lower risk of heart disease in later life. To give your baby a healthy start, eat a varied and well-balanced diet, including plenty of fresh fruit and vegetables and only a small intake of polyunsaturated fats. There is some evidence that mothers with elevated cholesterol levels could pass on problems to their unborn children, so it is important for these women to follow a heart-healthy diet and to see their doctors when planning a pregnancy.

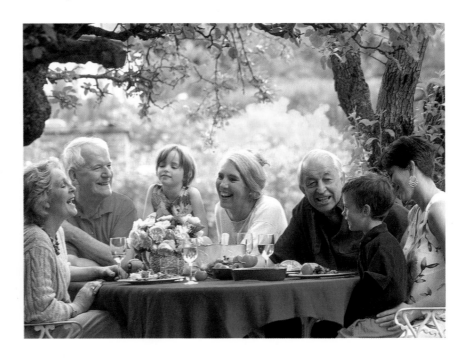

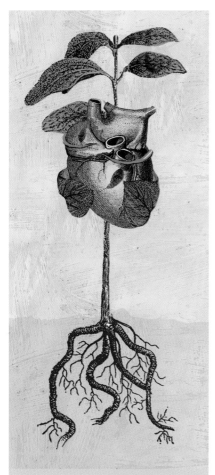

Protecting the heart

There is growing evidence to suggest that soy can help to reduce both total cholesterol and LDL cholesterol (by an average of 13 percent). Recently, the U.K. media reported that there is no evidence that genetically modified (GM) foods were harmful to health. GM soy has been made on a huge scale for some years in the United States.

products). As with any diet, however, there are good and bad ways of eating. A sensible vegetarian diet that is carefully planned and well balanced can meet all nutritional needs. In fact, it is often healthier than a meat-based diet, because it is lower in fat and higher in fiber. Encourage children thinking about becoming vegetarians to learn more about the subject and the importance of choosing a balanced diet that will benefit both their general and cardiovascular health.

Fruit and vegetables

Fruit and vegetables are heart-healthy for adults and children alike. Unfortunately, persuading children to eat vegetables is not always easy. Rather than trying to force them to eat vegetables they don't like, concentrate on those they will eat—colorful vegetables such as peas, carrots, and corn are often popular with kids. Children often prefer raw vegetables to cooked, so try adding a little grated carrot to salads or add some raw vegetables cut into fingers into their lunch boxes. Try sneaking vegetables into dishes such as spaghetti, casseroles, or pizza—Start by adding just a few at first, then gradually increase the amount.

JOIN CLUB MED

In some parts of Europe, the simple healthy eating principles outlined above are practiced as a way of life, with manifest benefits for

cardiovascular health. For example, the lowest rates of heart disease in Europe are found in countries around the Mediterranean.

The Mediterranean way

What's the secret of the Southern Europeans? Why are their hearts so much healthier than ours? The answer seems to lie in their culture of food—the things that they eat and the way that they eat them:

- The Mediterranean diet has a much higher ratio of poly-unsaturated and monounsaturated fats than the Northern European and North American diets; extra virgin olive oil, for example, is typically used in place of butter.
- People eat twice as much fruit and vegetables—six portions a day on average, the amount now recommended by U.S. doctors—boosting the level of antioxidants in the typical Mediterranean diet.
- Foods such as pasta, rice, fish, and salads are major features.
- Meals are a more central feature of daily life, which means that the Southern Europeans are more likely to sit down to a proper meal, cooked with fresh ingredients. They rely less on refined and processed "fast" food.

The combined result of these factors is to ensure a much more balanced diet that is naturally rich in complex carbohydrates, essential fatty acids, fiber and antioxidants, and low in saturated fat, salt, preservatives, and simple sugars.

People from Greece have just over two-thirds the risk of coronary heart disease of their Northern European and North American counterparts.

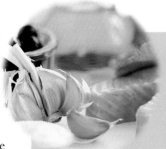

HEART-HEALTHY ATTITUDES

As we grow older our freedom to eat what and when we like can mean that our good habits can slip and bad habits develop. Parents do not always live by the healthy eating rules that they impose upon their children. Most parents would never send their child to school without a healthy brown-bag lunch, but they may not think twice about skipping lunch themselves or just snacking on a bag of chips. But there's no need for heart-healthy eating to be a chore, and it's well-worth making the effort to take a little care with your diet.

Quick heart foods

When time is tight, it can seem as though grabbing a burger or a bag of chips is the only option, but these can be damaging for your heart health. Here are a few time-saving ideas and meal suggestions to help you maintain healthy eating habits:

- Instead of running out to the newsstand or corner store for

HEART *SUPERFOODS*

Some foods can be singled out as being especially good for your heart. Eaten as part of a healthy balanced diet, these superfoods can improve your circulation and help to reduce blood pressure.

GARLIC As well as boosting "good" HDL cholesterol, garlic contains a substance—allicin—that helps to prevent and break down clots in the blood.

YOGURT A surprising addition, this dairy product is heart-friendly in small amounts; it's rich in calcium, which can help to correct high blood pressure.

OLIVE OIL In small doses, olive oil can help to reduce the tendency of blood to clot because it contains omega-6 fatty acids.

LEAFY VEGETABLES These contain plenty of fiber and the antioxidant chemicals beta-carotene and vitamin C.

OILY FISH Herring, mackerel, tuna, salmon, and sardines all contain fatty acids that boost HDL cholesterol, lower "bad" LDL cholesterol and reduce the risk of blood clots or thrombosis.

chocolate and chips, keep a supply of fresh and dried fruit at work to snack on when hunger strikes.

- Kebabs, whether fish, meat or vegetable, are quick to prepare and easy to cook. Brighten up your skewers with chunks of red onion, tomato, and sweet pepper and brush with a little Worcestershire sauce and olive oil.
- When you can't face cooking something complicated, try a simple stir fry. Just heat up a little olive oil in a

wok, toss in a generous portion of sliced vegetables, with some tangy ginger strips and crushed garlic; stir and serve with noodles.

- For a tasty dish, marinate fish (salmon works well), chicken, or pork overnight. Try a tangy mustard marinade: Mix together 2 level tablespoons of wholegrain mustard with 2 tablespoons each of apple juice and cider vinegar. When you get home, take the fish or meat out of the marinade and place on a hot grill for 10 minutes or until cooked. Serve with plenty of vegetables and a carbohydrate, such as pasta or potato.
- If you cook a healthy evening meal, such as a pasta salad, make a little extra for a brown-bag lunch the following day.

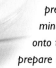

Heart-healthy meals in minutes
Simple dishes, such as fish brochettes, can be prepared in a matter of minutes and popped onto the grill while you prepare a salad and some couscous.

Maintaining weight and shape

Striking a balance between being too fat and too thin can mean the difference between a disease-free heart and smooth-running blood and a cardiovascular system under potentially life-threatening stress.

Being within the healthy weight range for your height is important for your cardiovascular health. If you are underweight, you may not be eating enough to provide your heart with the nutrients it needs to function properly. And if you are overweight, you could be putting your heart under stress. As body weight creeps up, so too does the risk of heart-related health problems.

A HEAVY HEART

Carrying excess weight increases the risk of several serious health problems, including heart disease, high blood pressure, and stroke. Obese women between the ages of 30 and 55 are seven times more likely to die from heart disease than women of the same age within the ideal weight range.

Check if you are a healthy weight using the body mass index (BMI) calculator on the right. A BMI between 18.5 and 25 is associated with the lowest heath risks. Risks increase slightly below 18.5 and increase significantly above 25, with a dramatic surge over 30.

APPLES AND PEARS

Your body composition—how much of your weight is fat and where that fat is stored—is an important factor in determining the health risks linked to being overweight. Your BMI doesn't give you this information, so you'll need to measure your waist to give you a better idea. If your BMI is over 25 and your waist measurement is more than 35 inches if you are a

woman or 41 inches for a man, then the excess weight you are carrying is more likely to be fat than muscle.

Fat stored around the waist—an apple-shaped body—is linked with health problems, particularly an increased risk of diabetes, heart disease, high blood pressure, and abnormal blood fat levels. Fat stored around the hips—a pear shape— seems to be less problematic.

Whether you're an apple or a pear tends to be influenced by your genes. Generally, men seem to carry their weight around their waists and women around their hips, putting men at greater risk of the problems associated with being overweight.

Calculating your BMI

Body Mass Index (BMI) is the most accurate predictor of whether your health is at risk because of your being overweight. The calculation has to be done using metric measurements.

BMI = *your weight in kilograms divided by your height in meters (squared).*

For example, Amanda weighs 132 pounds (60 kg) and is 5 feet 4 inches (1.65 m) tall. Her BMI is:

60 ÷ (1.65 x 1.65) = 22

Amanda's BMI of 22 places her squarely in the acceptable range, meaning that she is a healthy weight for her height.

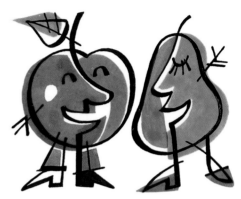

Are you a healthy shape?
It's better to be a pear than an apple when it comes to heart health. Weight carried around the abdomen increases the risk of a number of heart conditions.

Other factors, such as smoking and drinking alcohol, seem to increase the likelihood of fat being laid down around the stomach, while exercise helps to reduce body fat. The good news for apple-shapes is that it is easier to lose central fat than that stored around the hips. Whatever shape you are, losing any excess inches will benefit your heart.

LOSING WEIGHT SAFELY

There is no mystery to why we gain weight—It's a simple equation: When the energy (calories) we take in exceeds the energy we use, the excess is stored as fat. Eating just a small amount in excess of your needs will result in a slow, steady weight gain.

To lose weight, you simply need to tip the scale so that you use more calories than you consume—Your body will then draw on fat reserves to get the energy it needs. You can do this by restricting the number of calories you eat or by increasing the amount of calories you use, but without doubt the best way involves a combination of diet and exercise.

MENU *IDEAS FOR WEIGHT LOSS*

Just because you're cutting down on fat doesn't mean you have to cut down on taste. Whether you're counting calories or grams of fat, try the calculated meal ideas below for a successful weight-loss plan.

breakfast

- *High-fiber cereal with low-fat milk and a glass of orange juice = 350 kcal; 6 g fat.*
- *High-fiber banana muffin and low-fat yogurt with a glass of apple juice = 320 kcal; 7 g fat.*

lunch

- *A chicken drumstick, serving of broccoli, and a baked potato with cottage cheese = 400 kcal; 5.5 g fat.*
- *A chicken salad sandwich, using two slices of wholegrain bread, a small amount of low-fat spread, 2¾ ounces roast chicken and plenty of salad = 370 kcal; 14 g fat.*

dinner

- *Tofu, egg noodles, tomato sauce, bread with low-fat spread and a green salad dressed with olive oil = 500 kcal; 10 g fat.*
- *Grilled 5½ ounces of salmon fillet with 4 ounces of new potatoes and portion of ratatouille. About 500 kcal; 23 g fat.*

snacks and drinks

- *1¾ ounces ready-to-eat dried apricots = 80 kcal; 0.4 g fat.*
- *Banana smoothie made with small banana, one small container of low-fat yogurt and 3½ oz skim milk = 180 kcal; 1 g fat.*
- *Two pancakes with 1¾ oz cottage cheese = 180 kcal; 7 g fat.*
- *150 ml dry white wine = 150 kcal; 0 g fat.*
- *Apple juice (4 oz) = 60 kcal; 0 g fat.*
- *Orange juice (4 oz) = 60 kcal; 0 g fat.*
- *Cup of tea or coffee with low-fat milk = 11 kcal; 0.3 g fat.*

ALLOCATING YOUR CALORIES OR GRAMS

Use these rough guidelines to help break up your calories (kcal) or grams of fat across meals in a day. Refer to page 78 for the ideal daily calorie range for weight loss.

	1200 kcal	1500 kcal	44 g fat	55 g fat
Breakfast	300 kcal	300 kcal	11 g	11 g
Lunch	350 kcal	400 kcal	13 g	15 g
Dinner	400 kcal	500 kcal	14 g	18 g
Snacks	150 kcal	300 kcal	6 g	11 g

Diet dilemmas

Unfortunately when it comes to losing weight, there are no miracle cures or quick fixes. How often have you been tempted by the promise of losing 7 pounds in seven days, only to find that the very next week you've regained all the weight you lost plus a little more? Crash diets, however tempting they sound, are not the answer. Although you may lose weight initially, the chances are you'll end up putting it all back on. If you need to lose weight, what you really need to do is change your eating habits on a long-term basis.

Yo-yo dieting—repeatedly losing and regaining weight—is not healthy. The best and safest way to lose weight is slowly and steadily; an ideal rate is 1 to 2 pounds a week. If you lose too much weight too quickly, there's a danger that you'll also lose lean muscle tissue. Since your metabolic rate is related to the amount of lean muscle tissue you have, it's a good idea to do whatever you can to preserve it.

A life-long commitment

Don't think about dieting as a short-term solution—The only way to lose weight safely and permanently is to make long-term changes in your food choices, eating habits, and lifestyle. Forget about dieting; think about a whole new way of eating. The good

> *Eating just 100 calories a day more than you need—the equivalent of two or three cookies—will result in a weight gain of 10 pounds in a year.*

news is that this doesn't have to mean missing out on your favorite foods; in fact, it's important to include the foods you enjoy eating. A diet that leaves you feeling deprived, unhappy, and dissatisfied is a diet that will quickly be abandoned.

To achieve steady, healthy weight loss, you need to reduce your normal calorie intake by around 600 calories a day. For most women, an intake of 1200 to 1500 calories a day should be sufficient, and 1750 to 1950 calories should work for men. It's important that you spread your allowance throughout the whole day—Eating little and often will help you to maintain a steady blood sugar level and reduce the temptation to snack or binge.

Whatever diet plan you choose to follow, the basic principle will be the same—Eat fewer calories. Because fat contains twice as many calories as either protein or carbohydrate, the most effective way of reducing your calorie intake is to keep the amount of fat you eat to a sensible minimum.

PREVENTING MIDDLE-AGE WEIGHT GAIN

Putting on weight does not need to be an inevitable part of growing older. Although our resting metabolic rates decline with age—a reduction of about 5 percent each decade—the effect is modest. A 40-year-old woman, for example, would burn 70 fewer calories a day than a 30-year-old woman. A more likely reason for middle-age weight gain is that our levels of physical activity decrease rapidly with age. If energy intake is not reduced to match, excess energy will be stored in the body as fat.

Small steps to diet success

Simple changes, such as switching from whole milk to low-fat milk, using low-fat spread instead of butter, and cutting out sugar in tea and coffee will all help to prevent middle-age weight gain. Just as important as the foods you choose is the way you prepare them. Always use cooking methods that involve little or no fat. See page 67 for ideas on how to trim the fat from your diet.

Get active

Exercise preserves and develops muscle tissue, which is metabolically more active than fat—muscle uses more calories—so that the more muscle you have, the more calories your body burns. Exercise can also help to improve your body shape and is good for all-around heart health.

Small changes in routine such as walking part of the way to work or running up the stairs rather than taking the elevator all increase energy expenditure. The secret is to build exercise into your daily routine. Find activities you enjoy that fit in with your lifestyle, and be realistic—Start slowly and gradually build up the frequency and length of time you exercise. For more information on getting into shape and some great exercise ideas for heart health, see the following section, pages 80 to 88.

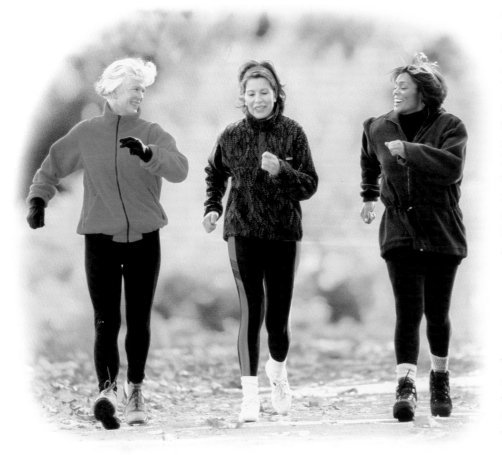

Walk your way to a healthier heart
Increasing the amount of exercise you get is one of the easiest ways to ensure you lose excess weight. Walking, whether outside or on a treadmill in a gym, is great exercise.

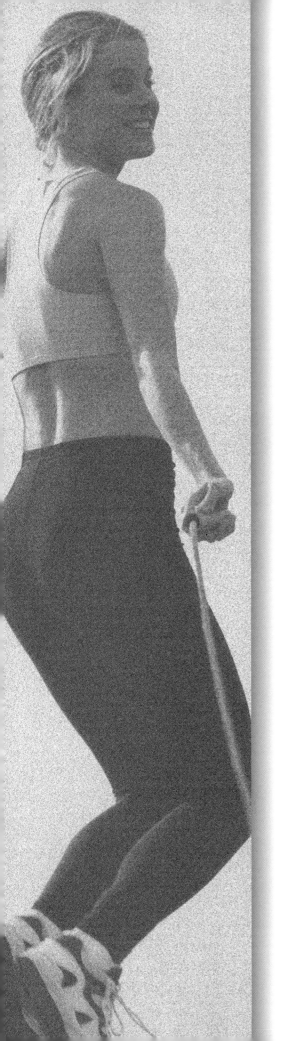

EXERCISE YOUR HEART

Physical activity helps you to make the most of life. It can give you energy and make you feel better, adding years to your life and life to your years. Just like any other muscle, your heart needs exercise to keep it in good shape. Exercising regularly, at a suitable intensity, makes your heart stronger and better able to cope with its relentless task of pumping blood around the body. For maximum effect, choose activities that suit your age, current physical condition, and lifestyle.

Regular aerobic exercise gives your heart a welcome workout and can make a real difference to your heart health.

You don't have to take up a new sport to keep fit. Simply being more active in your everyday life can be enough.

Gradually increase the intensity of your exercise once you're fit. Remember to warm up before starting and cool down afterward.

Once you're exercising regularly, assess your progress and fitness. Monitor your pulse to check that you're exercising effectively.

Exercise benefits for your heart

Exercise is good for your heart; there's no denying it. Having an active life dramatically reduces your risk of heart disease and stroke—two of the biggest killers in the Western world; what's more, it can help you to feel better and live longer.

Physical inactivity is among the worst risk factors for coronary heart disease— It is a little behind smoking but has an impact similar to that of high cholesterol and blood pressure. In addition to slashing the risk of heart disease and stroke, regular exercise lowers your blood pressure and brings about favorable changes in your cholesterol levels.

THE SEDENTARY LIFESTYLE

The heart does not thrive inside an inert body. Sitting all day, driving to the supermarket, and using leisure time to watch television, visit the movies, or go to a restaurant, all constitute a sedentary lifestyle. This sort of exercise-free existence is all too common and is bad news for your heart. According to a Harvard study, 60 percent of adults in the United States do not get enough exercise in their lives. Sedentary people have nearly twice the risk of a fatal heart attack as active people of the same age. If the sedentary lifestyle sounds familiar, then it is time to make some changes to give your heart a chance.

GO AEROBIC!

The word "aerobic" comes from the Greek meaning "with air." In exercise terms, it means any activity that raises the heart rate, by moving the large muscles of the legs (and arms) continuously for extended periods of time. Aerobic exercise is the best for cardiovascular health.

With regular aerobic activity, the body becomes more efficient at extracting oxygen from the blood. The heart becomes stronger and pumps more blood in a single stroke with fewer beats per minute—which explains why pulse rate is a useful measure of fitness (see pages 90 to 91).

(see pages 90 to 91).

IT'S NOT TRUE!

"A fit-looking body equals a fit heart"

Just because someone looks in great shape on the outside, it doesn't mean that hir or her heart is in the same good condition. Muscle-building exercises to tone and strengthen muscles are anaerobic—meaning "without air"—so don't give the heart a workout. Aerobic exercise is needed to promote heart health.

WORKING THE MUSCLE

The heart is a muscle like any other, and as such it requires exercise to enable it to function efficiently. Without the stimulation of aerobic physical activity, the heart shrinks, so it can't hold enough blood and doesn't have the muscle power for a strong contraction.

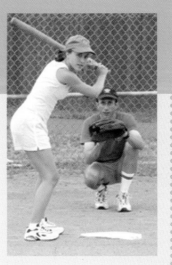

IT'S NEVER TOO LATE TO START EXERCISING

By exercising regularly at moderate intensity for 30 minutes on five or more days a week, you will be rewarded with more and more benefits for your heart health over a relatively short time.

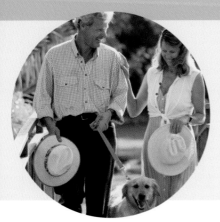

1 TO 2 WEEKS
Your heart muscle has begun to strengthen, and its blood supply is already increasing. Your circulation has improved, and more oxygen is carried by the blood to the tissues.

1 MONTH
You may notice significant changes in your energy level. Your resting heart rate is now slower than before you started exercising, and your blood contains more red blood cells.

Performing regular aerobic exercise can lower diastolic blood pressure by about 5 percent over 12 weeks.

With a little training, the heart muscle becomes much more efficient, enlarges slightly, and can rest longer between beats.

IMPROVING CIRCULATION

Your whole circulatory system benefits from exercise. As your heart works faster, your blood vessels benefit, too. During an aerobic exercise session, the volume of the liquid part of blood—the plasma—rises, diluting the concentration of the oxygen-carrying hemoglobin in red blood cells. Blood then flows through the blood vessels faster and more freely, the return of blood to the heart is faster, and the volume of blood passing through it in a single beat is greater. Improved blood flow lowers the risk of ischemia—in which insufficient blood and oxygen reaches the body tissues—and of peripheral vascular disease.

LOWERING BLOOD PRESSURE

Frequent aerobic exercise—about 30 minutes five times a week—reduces blood pressure. With regular, sustained activity, muscles around the body grow in strength and size, and in order to supply them with oxygen and glucose the number of capillaries feeding the muscles increases to meet demand. By causing the formation of new tiny blood vessels, known as revascularization, exercise helps to lower blood pressure as the blood is distributed through a larger circulatory network.

LOWERING CHOLESTEROL

Regular aerobic exercise not only promotes levels of the "good" high-density lipoprotein (HDL) cholesterol but also lowers levels of the "bad" low-density lipoprotein (LDL) cholesterol. The overall action of exercise is to improve the balance between the two, shifting the all-important HDL to LDL ratio toward a healthier value.

CONTROLLING WEIGHT

Being overweight places the heart under great pressure and is a major risk factor for coronary artery disease. In conjunction with a weight-loss diet, exercise can help you shed excess pounds. Making aerobic exercise a regular part of your life will help you to keep to a healthy weight by burning excess calories and regulating your appetite.

STAYING YOUNG

It's never too late to start, but the sooner you do the better. By beginning gently and increasing your activity gradually, you can actually slow the physical process of aging. Researchers have discovered that people who are physically active have a biological age much less than their chronological age—proof that keeping fit keeps you young.

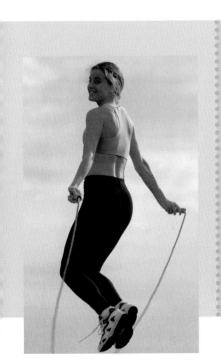

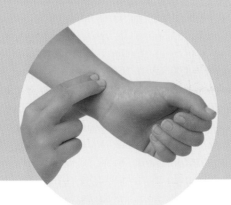

3 MONTHS
Your plasma lipid profile has improved, and your blood pressure has decreased, both while active and at rest. Your body is now fully adapted to the level of activity you have chosen, so you can consider increasing the intensity now.

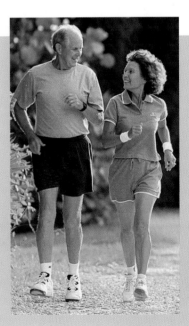

Build activity into your life

How much better off will your heart be as a result of being more active on a day-to-day basis? Significantly, is the answer. Halving your risk of heart disease starts with simply ensuring your heart gets enough exercise most days.

The way you live can make a real difference to the health of your heart. We have all heard about the studies that show that an active lifestyle drastically reduces the risk of developing heart disease. But many of us equate being active with images of people working out at the gym or taking part in structured sports or exercise several days of the week. Sometimes it's difficult to see how this could fit into our own lives.

A NEW LOOK AT ACTIVITY

Becoming more physically active doesn't have to involve much effort on your part or change from your usual commitments. Try examining what you do in your daily life and see if you could do things differently to increase your amount of physical activity. For example, why drive to the supermarket for a missing ingredient for a meal, when it can be almost as quick—and much better for your heart—to walk or cycle?

Studies back the active life

Recent studies have shown that it is being active on a day-to-day basis that is the determining factor in your cardiovascular health.

One such study in the United States followed 235 people, half of whom regularly attended supervised exercise sessions while the other half incorporated 30 minutes of moderately intense activity into their daily routines. After six months, the group getting

Thirty is the magic number
Clock up your activity minutes to 30 minutes a day. Whether you love gardening or lavish attention on your home, it's good to know that your heart benefits at the same time.

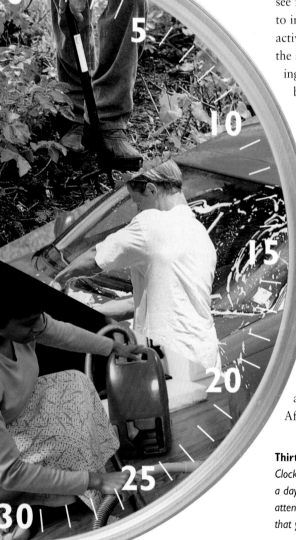

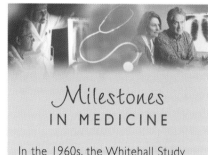

Milestones
IN MEDICINE

In the 1960s, the Whitehall Study on the health of UK civil servants found that low-grade workers were three times more likely to die from heart disease than those in higher grades. This was partly because they were more likely to smoke and less likely to exercise regularly, but factors such as work stress may also have contributed.

structured exercise showed greater improvements in cardiovascular fitness than the "lifestyle" group. However, after two years both sets of participants were found to be significantly more active than they were to start with and experienced improved cardiovascular health and exercise performance.

HOW MUCH IS ENOUGH?

Experts agree that we should aim for about 30 minutes of moderately intense activity on at least five days of the week. But how does this translate into your normal routine? An easily accessible definition of moderately intense activity is anything that leaves you feeling warm and slightly out of breath.

Break it up

Sometimes it can seem like setting aside a whole 30 minutes for an activity is just not feasible. However, you don't have to do it all in one

A Japanese study found that people who have a 20-minute walk to work each day have half the risk of heart disease compared with those whose walk takes 10 minutes.

session. Three 10-minute sessions of activity during the day will also produce cardiovascular health benefits, so try breaking down your activity into smaller chunks if that fits more easily in with your lifestyle.

If your current level of physical activity is low, this is an excellent springboard to start getting your heart into gear and get it well on the way to health and fitness.

So if it's just a case of introducing activity into your life for 30 minutes a day, what's stopping you?

Plan your week

Spend some time thinking through your day or week—and then plan things that you can do to become more active. Many people find that a few minutes spent thinking about which type of activity suits them and when they can fit it into their schedule pays dividends.

Don't assume that a healthy level of activity will automatically disrupt your everyday life—With a sensible approach it will actually enhance it, and your heart will thank you.

Add up your activities

Activities that fit easily into your daily routine are more likely to be sustained in the long term. Don't forget do-it-yourself (DIY) household activities. One way of checking if you are meeting the daily 30-minute quota of moderately intense activity is to add up the number of calories you have used in different activities. A weekly total of 2000 calories (kcal) or more will ensure an impact on your cardiovascular health.

KCAL /MIN	ACTIVITY
3	Dusting
3	Walking (2 mph)
4	Cycling (6 mph)
4	DIY (light e.g. decorating)
4	Gardening (light)
4	Mopping floor
4	Walking (4 mph)
4	Vacuuming
6	DIY (moderate e.g. carpentry)
6	Polishing furniture
6	Scrubbing floor
7	Cycling (10 mph)
8	DIY (heavy e.g. cement mixing)
8	Gardening (digging)
9	Cycling (12 mph)

Count the minutes you spend on each activity; then multiply by the appropriate number of kilocalories per minute to calculate the number of calories you have used.

EXAMPLE: TOM'S WEEKLY ACTIVITY RECORD

Tom has a 25-minute brisk walk as part of his commute to work each day (50 min x 5 days x 4 kcal/min =1000 kcal).

On the weekend, Tom gardens for a couple of hours (120 min x 4 kcal/min = 480 kcal).

He mops the kitchen floor (20 min x 4 kcal/min = 80 kcal) and vacuums (30 min x 4 kcal/min = 120 kcal).

On Sunday, Tom decides to cycle to the garden center instead of taking the car (2 x 20 min x 9 kcal/min = 360 kcal).

During this week, Tom has burned 2040 kcal—easily enough to keep his heart healthy.

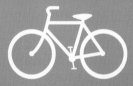

CYCLE TO HEART HEALTH

Cycling is a great way of keeping active and exercising your heart. It requires rhythmic effort of the aerobic nature your heart needs.

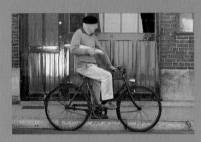

Take a ride into town to do your shopping, instead of hopping on a bus or getting in the car.

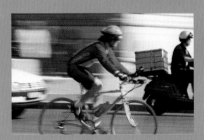

Get into the habit of cycling to work, and make use of the growing number of cycle routes.

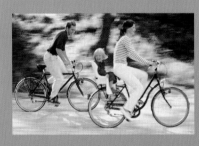

Cycling can be incorporated into most day-to-day life—including trips out with the family.

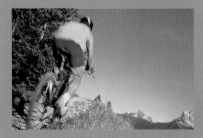

Variable wind speeds and changes in gradient mean that your body needs to work at a variety of rates.

NO TIME TO BE ACTIVE? EXCUSES, EXCUSES . . .

A U.S. survey showed that the most common reason that people do not exercise is a lack of time, but when we have to find only 30 minutes a day, there really are no excuses. For many people, work and family grab the majority of their time, but it should be easy to revitalize your heart by incorporating more physical activity into this time.

HAVE YOURSELF SOME FAMILY FUN

A full family life can mean that you have little time or energy left at the end of a day. But why not use your family time constructively to become more active? Not only will the activity benefit your heart, but also your children's—and they'll appreciate the quality time that shared exercise provides. You will also be presenting a good role model for the next generation to follow.

WORKOUT AROUND WORK

Full-time work can sometimes seem to take up most of your energy and leave you with little leisure time, so you need to sneak in some activity wherever you can. There are plenty of opportunities to be active as you go about your day-to-day work.

Use the stairs to get to your office instead of using the elevator: It is excellent exercise for your legs and your heart.

When you take the kids to the park, take along a ball for a game, and join in the fun yourself.

Try walking or cycling at least some of the way to work; get off two bus stops earlier or park your car further away. Or combine a folding bicycle with public transportation.

Make use of any plans your company offers for reduced-price admission to local sports clubs.

At lunchtime, take a brisk walk in the park with colleagues.

Walk the children to school instead of using the car; you could offer to pick up their friends, too, along the way.

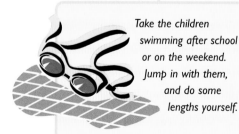

Take the children swimming after school or on the weekend. Jump in with them, and do some lengths yourself.

Cycle into town as a family to go shopping on the weekend. Investigate safe cycle routes, and be sure your children are safe cyclists first.

Give your heart a workout

Taking up an exercise program is a great way to ensure you keep your heart fit. Whatever exercise you choose, be sure to work out safely by always incorporating the three essential stages: warming up, working out, and cooling down.

Getting your heart fit means leaving behind sedentary ways. Enjoying being active—playing in the office softball team or enjoying a round of golf on the weekend—is a step in the right direction. Once you've seen how easy and fun it can be to include activity in your daily routine, a logical step is to increase your level of exercise to boost your heart's potential further.

Remind yourself of the benefits of exercise and how soon you'll reap the rewards of extra fitness. But remember that what you get back depends on how much you put in.

STARTING OUT
Most people under age 45 are fit enough to begin exercising at a moderate level of intensity, but for everyone the best advice is to start slowly and progress gradually. If you want to start more structured exercise, or to increase the level of sports you do, then it may be worthwhile to check with your doctor first (see page 48). You should always consult your doctor if you have had heart trouble in the past, have high blood pressure, or are prone to dizziness or fainting.

A FITT FRAME OF MIND
There are four aspects of exercise to consider when beginning a structured program: frequency, intensity, time, and type.

Frequency
How often can you exercise? Ideally you should exercise four or five days per week. If you have been fairly sedentary, it is all the more

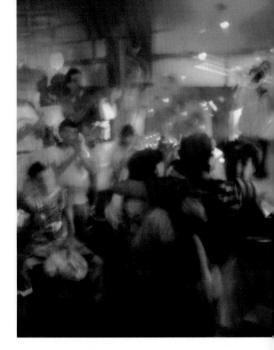

Dancing for a heart workout
You don't always have to go out jogging or running to exercise your heart. An evening dancing can provide a good aerobic workout if you keep it up long enough!

important that you exercise as frequently as possible because you will not be able to exercise intensively or for prolonged periods.

Intensity
How energetic can you be? This will depend on your existing level of fitness. It's best to start with low-intensity exercise—defined as a level that equals 50 to 60 percent of your maximal heart rate (see page 91). If you are already fit and getting exercise, you may be able to exercise at a higher intensity.

Time
How long can you set aside for each session? You don't always have to devote the same length of time to each session. On some days you may be able to set aside more time than others. If you do an activity that is very intensive, you probably won't want to spend as long doing it as you would it you did a less intensive activity.

Exercise—how aerobic is it?

For an effective heart workout, choose activities that are 50 percent aerobic or more—Here are some examples, and you may be in for a few surprises.

%	ACTIVITY
100	Jogging, long-distance running
95	Cross-country skiing
90	Brisk walking (3–4 mph)
80	2-mile run; vigorous cycling; aerobic dancing
75	800 m swim (32 lengths)
65	1-mile run, football, active social dancing
60	Rowing (2 km)
50	Heavy gardening or digging
25	Tennis
15	100 m swim (4 lengths), squash

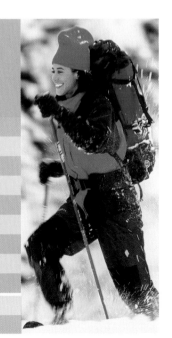

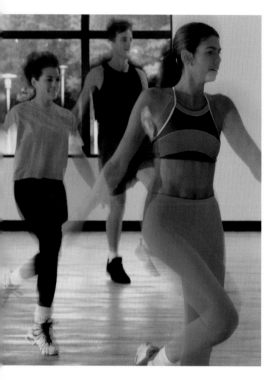

Don't rush in
Before any exercise, take time to warm up: Five minutes spent running around a football field before putting all your energies into a game raises your pulse rate and warms your muscles, making them less prone to injury.

Type

What kind of activities do you enjoy? You are more likely to remain motivated and continue your exercise program if you do activities you like. If you are a regular exerciser, then you need to examine the type of activity you're doing to give your heart a workout. Playing tennis once a week may keep you supple and strong, but all that stopping and starting means it's not very aerobic (see the chart on page 85) and so isn't the ideal exercise for improving your heart's fitness. Think about adding an aerobic exercise such as running, swimming, or cycling.

SAFETY FIRST

Whether you work out regularly or are new to exercise, following safety guidelines is important—You need to ease your body into your aerobic workout, monitor yourself in action, and allow your body to cool down. Knowing how to manage and maintain your activity level is the key to exercising for a fit heart.

WARMING UP

Before taking part in any activity, it is important that you take the time to warm up. There are inherent dangers in rushing into exercise without first preparing your heart and muscles for the job that lies ahead; your body may not be able to meet the demands you are making on it, and you could end up feeling stiff, sore, and exhausted.

Warming up should include both gentle pulse-raising activities for the heart and gentle stretching exercises for the muscles and joints.

There are very good reasons for warming the body up before beginning any exercise:

- When the body temperature is raised, the oxygen being carried in the blood is released more easily, making more energy available, so you perform better and do not tire so quickly. You should aim to warm up for 5 to 10 minutes, gradually increasing your pulse rate until you feel slightly warmer and are breathing more deeply.

- When your muscles are warm, they can contract more easily, and flexibility can be improved by more than 20 percent. This greater range of movement within the joints means that ligaments and tendons are far less likely to be damaged, thus preventing injury.

In some activities, you can simply apply the warming-up principle to the first five minutes of your session. For example, if you are running, take it easy initially to get your heart rate up and your muscles warm; the same goes for taking it easy for the last five or ten minutes to cool down.

When working out, your heart can pump an incredible seven times the volume of blood as it does when resting.

positive health tips

Exercise safely

In order to avoid injury, follow these health and safety tips:

- Start slowly and progress gradually—Set realistic aims.

- Warm up and cool down before and after each session.

- Be aware of the environment: Wear a hat and gloves in cold weather, and don't overdo it when it's hot.

- Don't exercise after a large meal or after consuming alcohol.

- Listen to your body.

- Don't exercise hard if you have a cold or other infection.

If you feel unwell while you are exercising, stop immediately and take it easier next time.

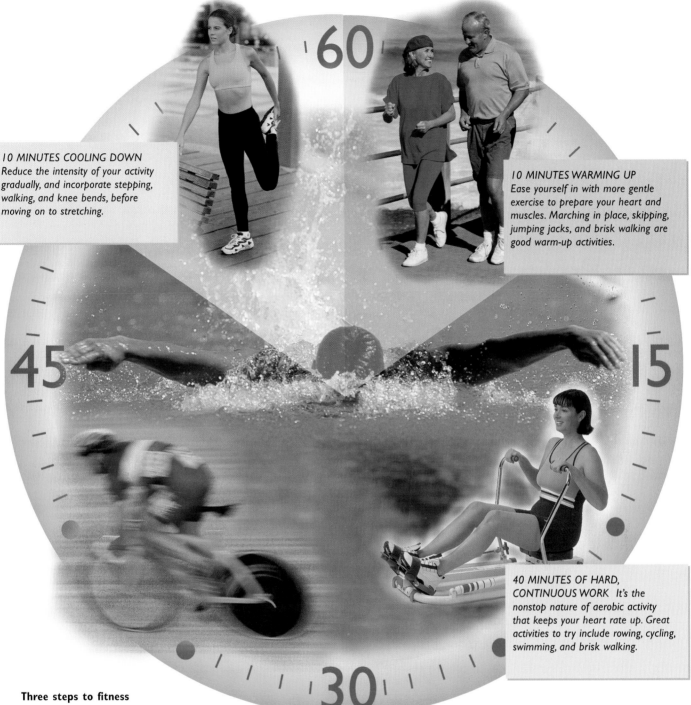

10 MINUTES COOLING DOWN
Reduce the intensity of your activity gradually, and incorporate stepping, walking, and knee bends, before moving on to stretching.

10 MINUTES WARMING UP
Ease yourself in with more gentle exercise to prepare your heart and muscles. Marching in place, skipping, jumping jacks, and brisk walking are good warm-up activities.

40 MINUTES OF HARD, CONTINUOUS WORK *It's the nonstop nature of aerobic activity that keeps your heart rate up. Great activities to try include rowing, cycling, swimming, and brisk walking.*

Three steps to fitness
Whether you go swimming on your lunch hour, jogging in the evening, or to the gym on the weekend, remember to ease yourself gently into and out of your exercise session.

WORKING OUT

Start at an intensity level that you will be able to continue comfortably for 30 to 40 minutes; after a few weeks, you'll find you can start to push yourself a little harder. Your heart benefits more from a longer moderate workout than a faster shorter one. To assess whether you are exercising safely as well as effectively, remember to listen to what your body is telling you.

• Your heart should be beating faster than usual, but not racing.

• You should be breathing more deeply and more rapidly, but not out of control—if you can talk to someone easily while exercising, you are working at the right level.

• You should be warm and sweaty during exercise, but not dripping.

Be careful to increase the length and intensity of your exercise gradually. If you experience any uncomfortable

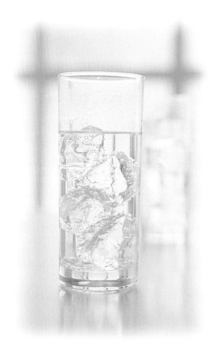

stiffness or pain following activity then you have overdone things, so ease off a little next time.

You should find that your fitness builds quickly, which will give you the energy to enjoy life to the fullest.

Regulate yourself

It is always good to measure your progress throughout your exercise program. Seeing improvements in your fitness is a great motivator to keep going. There are easy ways to tell if you are becoming more fit. Are you completing your normal walk, run, or cycle in less time? Are you less out of breath and able to exercise easier? Does your pulse rate return quickly to normal when you have finished exercising? If your answers are yes, then you are obviously reaping the benefits of your exercise program.

Cool down and stretch out
Spend 5 to 10 minutes cooling down and then 5 minutes stretching. Your muscles are still warm, and stretching is a great way to increase their flexibility and suppleness.

Stay hydrated
Vigorous aerobic exercise produces more heat, so you will sweat more easily as your body attempts to keep your temperature constant. Replace the fluid lost during training by sipping water throughout your session.

Staying hydrated

It is essential that you drink plenty of fluids before and during exercise, to prevent dehydration. The body can lose an amazing 2 to 3 quarts of water per hour through sweat. If you are exercising for a prolonged period of time, consider using isotonic sports drinks, which replace salts and sugar as well as water. These drinks provide energy and prevent dehydration.

COOLING DOWN

Regardless of the type of exercise you choose, a cooling down period of five to ten minutes is essential. When you are active, all the blood vessels in your body open up to aid circulation to the muscles, which then squeeze blood to the heart. If you stop suddenly and just stand still with vessels still dilated, the heart has difficulty keeping up the supply to some areas without the help of the muscles. Gravity drains the blood away from the brain, and you are liable to feel dizzy or faint.

At the end of your session of activity, you should allow yourself roughly 10 to 15 minutes to cool down and to stretch those muscles that you have been using.

- Gradually slow the pace of the activity you are doing and reduce the intensity. For example, if you are running, slow down to a jog for five minutes and then a walk.
- Include some flexibility exercises. Go through a series of stretches, trying to hold each stretch for 30 seconds. Never force your body to stretch more than is comfortable, and never bounce during a stretch. In addition to increasing flexibility, stretching can prevent you from feeling stiff the following day.

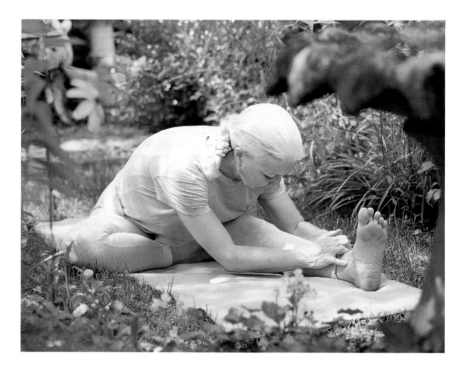

Maximizing your potential

If you want to push yourself to the peak of cardiovascular fitness, a few simple techniques can help you monitor your improvements and make sure you work at the right level— not too hard but hard enough—for heart health.

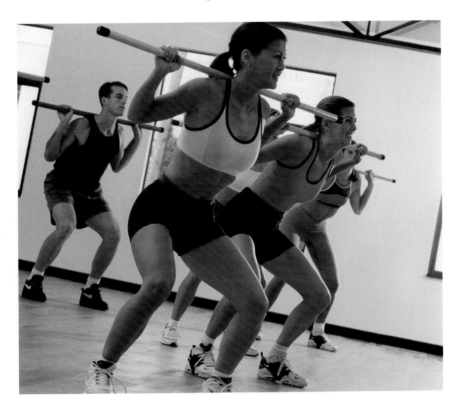

You probably experienced some positive mental benefits after your first exercise session. And after exercising regularly for 10 to 12 weeks, you should really feel the physical benefits of your efforts: You'll have more energy for day-to-day life, and you'll feel less breathless during exercise and recover more quickly after a session. By this stage, exercise will have become a firm part of your weekly routine; but then what?

ACHIEVING MORE
Having made the time and given the commitment to exercise, you have to push yourself each time to continue to improve your heart's fitness. Why not try adding a weekly circuit

Working harder
Try joining a more strenuous exercise class once a week to increase your fitness. Classes that combine weights with aerobic exercise help you to work your body harder.

training session or a step class as an extra dimension, or take up a new sport? You are ready to start a more demanding exercise regime and may even wish to start taking part in competitive events.

Changing goals
Initially, you may start out wanting to improve your heart health but, as your fitness level improves, find you want to strive for your own physical

potential. It's not unusual for your fitness goals to change with improved fitness; since now everything you do in life seems to take less effort, it is only natural to want to do more. Three months into your aerobic program, your body will be ready for a more exacting challenge.

A FINGER ON THE PULSE
Measuring your pulse rate is an excellent way to monitor improvements in your fitness and can also help you to make changes to your personal training program. Your pulse is an indirect way of measuring your heart rate, usually done in beats per minute (bpm). If you took your pulse rate when you first started exercising, you should notice how much your resting value has fallen as your heart has become stronger and more efficient at pumping blood around your body.

Keep the pressure on
Your pulse rate during and after exercise provides an accurate index of how hard your heart is working. Without monitoring your pulse, you can actually become less fit. As your body adapts to the demands of the exercise program, you find it physically easier; you may find you are no longer making enough demands on your heart to increase your fitness. Without being aware of this, you can gradually decondition. The pulse rate indicates if you are working hard enough—it also warns you if you are doing too much.

After a break
Monitoring your pulse rate is particularly important if you start exercising again after a long period of physical inactivity. Sports

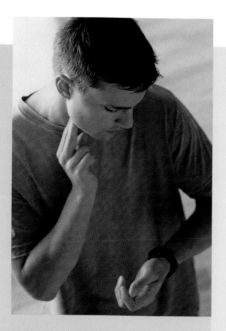

Monitoring pulse recovery time
How quickly your pulse returns to its resting value after a session is a great indicator of your heart's fitness. The more fit you become, the faster your heart recovers. Take a reading every minute to track your recovery time.

GET THE MOST FROM YOUR EXERCISE PROGRAM

To maximize your heart's fitness, push yourself to work within your target heart rate zone. You can work out your own training zone from a formula. First, subtract your age from the number 220; then calculate 60 to 80 percent of the number you end up with. For ease, you can refer to the chart opposite.

How to take your pulse

There are pulse points all over your body, but only a couple are accessible for measurement during exercise: the carotid pulse in your neck and the radial pulse at your wrist. Taking your pulse accurately is a skill you learn with practice, and it can quickly become a routine part of your exercise program. First

of all, position yourself where you can see a clock with a second hand, or use a wristwatch. Stop briefly—for 15 seconds—when you are actually measuring your pulse.

- For your radial pulse, place the fore and middle fingers of one hand on the inside of the other wrist, just down from the base of the thumb. You may find that you need to move your fingers around a little until you can clearly feel the pulse.
- For your carotid pulse, using the same fingers place them on your neck just under your jawbone and press to feel a strong pulse.

While looking at the second hand of the clock or watch, count the number of heart beats you can feel

scientists have discovered that we lose cardiovascular fitness quicker than muscular fitness. In fact, after only two weeks of rest, there are significant reductions in aerobic capacity. So we may think that we can take part in quite vigorous activity when the heart and lungs are, in fact, not up to it. By taking your pulse to see how fit or unfit your heart has become, you can avoid overstressing it. Building up your activity slowly will allow your heart and lungs to "catch up" with the condition of your muscles.

MODIFYING YOUR ACTIVITY

To maintain a healthy level of cardiovascular fitness, you have to be active for life. Being athletic or exercising regularly in your youth is

a good start but provides no guarantee of future health benefits. However, your life may not always run so smoothly, and you may have to take a break from activity, for any number of reasons. This break

Competitive athletes have a resting pulse as low as about 40 beats per minute.

may be because of time pressures at work, a change in life circumstances, or recovery from illness or injury.

Just because you have to give up running or sports temporarily, it doesn't mean that you can't keep your heart fit. Try to think of

alternative ways of clocking 30 minutes of activity a day until you can get back to your original level of activity (see page 83). Walking is one of the best, most convenient and effective ways of maintaining your heart health and easing your body back into exercise after a break. Plan a number of walking routes that vary in length from 5 to 30 minutes and that you can do from your home. You will then be able to choose a route to suit the time you have available or how you are feeling.

Stepping down

All the changes you have worked so hard to gain—the improvement in the tone of your heart muscle, your body's ability to use oxygen efficiently, your lower resting pulse—

in 15 seconds. (If you counted for a whole minute, your heart would be slowing down all that time, and the pulse rate would be inaccurate.) Multiply the number of beats you count by four in order to obtain the number of heart beats per minute.

An alternative to measuring your own pulse is to wear a heart-rate monitor that is linked to a wristwatch: This monitor tells you at a glance how many beats a minute your heart is pumping.

Target heart rate zones
Your maximum heart rate will decrease as you get older. Exercise safely but effectively and try to stick within your effective heart rate zone. Follow the line up from your age to find your target heart rate.

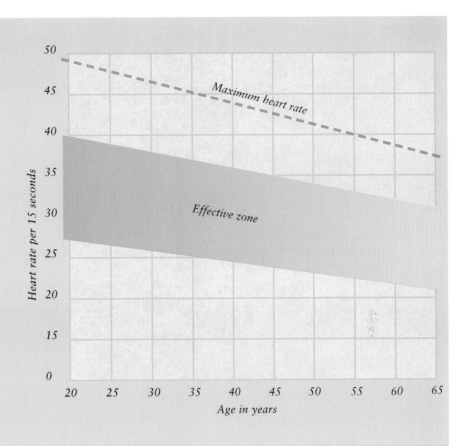

need not be lost. Rather than stopping an activity completely, you may be able to reduce the intensity at which you exercise or the amount of time you work out.

Following an injury

If you have sustained an injury or are recovering from an illness, be sensible. Don't expect to start exercising at your former level of intensity. Your body will have lost some of its fitness and you may expose it to further strain. Instead, listen to your body and learn to recognize the signs that indicate you are working at the correct intensity. Try a shorter or less intense workout, choose a non-weight-bearing activity—Swimming or cycling are both great alternatives.

Swimming is excellent for the heart, provided you complete a sufficient number of lengths (see page 85), as well as for mobility of major joints. It supports the body's weight and is ideal when a weight-bearing activity would be detrimental. Hydrotherapy is often used to regain cardiovascular fitness after certain illnesses or for people with certain conditions, such as arthritis.

Walking wonderland
A walking program may lead to a more ambitious and rewarding activity, such as hill walking. Exercising with others is a great motivator, too.

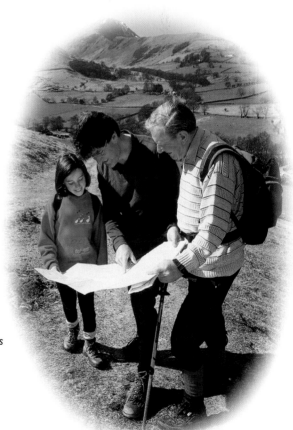

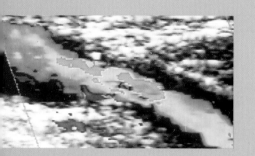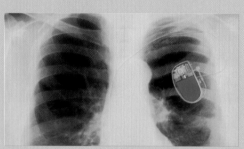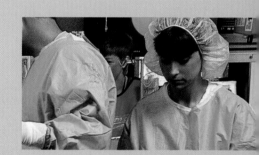

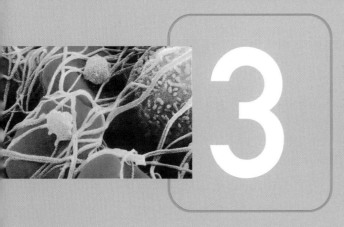

3

What happens
when things go wrong

Knowing what can go wrong

To fulfill the body's unrelenting needs, the heart demands a regular supply of fuel and electrical power, and its working parts must be fully functioning. Sometimes, for any variety of reasons, a fault develops in one of these areas that affects the smooth running of this vital organ.

GENETIC AND HEREDITARY FACTORS

Although the human genome project is almost complete, some work still remains to be done. However, experts have been able to prove that genes are the cause of particular diseases or abnormalities. Heart disease tends to run in families, as does high blood pressure—One positive aspect of this is that it enables early screening of people who are potentially at higher risk. For example, if one or both parents have coronary artery disease, their children have an increased risk of developing the condition in later life. The common condition of varicose

heart, giving the baby a bluish tinge around the mouth and fingers. Not so long ago, babies with serious congenital conditions would inevitably die. Today, surgery can often repair the defect successfully.

Many congenital abnormalities are comparatively minor, and some even disappear naturally as the baby grows. "Holes in the heart" are defects in the walls, or septa, that divide the left side of the heart from the right side of the heart, and vary in severity. In mild cases, these conditions may only come to light during a routine medical examination in adult life.

MORE COMMON

HYPERTENSION	INTERMITTENT CLAUDICATION	VARICOSE VEINS	DILATED CARDIOMYOPATHY
Hypertension affects 25 percent of people living in North America.	*5 percent of men and 2.5 percent of women 60 years or older*	*50 percent of adults; twice as prevalent in women as in men.*	*1 per 50*
ATHEROSCLEROSIS	HEART ATTACK		
Every adult in the Western world has a degree of atherosclerosis.	*1.1 million each year*	ANGINA	
		About 4 million people in the United States suffer from angina.	

veins characteristically runs in families, as does the rarer disease hypertrophic cardiomyopathy, which causes muscle in the wall of the left chamber of the heart to thicken. In certain cases, one or more of the heart valves, which keep the blood flowing in one direction in the heart, are faulty because of an abnormal gene.

CONGENITAL CONDITIONS

The development of the heart in the embryo is a complicated process, and it is not surprising that occasionally things go wrong and babies are born with abnormal hearts. Sometimes, a heart abnormality is complex, with more than one structure involved. For example, an affected baby may have a combination of a "hole in the heart," abnormal valves, and the wrong artery coming out of a ventricle. Deoxygenated blood on its way to the lungs may be diverted to the left side of the

AT THE LEADING EDGE

New risk factors for heart disease

Exactly why the coronary arteries become narrowed remains the subject of high-profile medical research. Most people are aware of the classic risk factors—smoking, high cholesterol, and lack of exercise. New risk factors, however, are still being identified. The levels of certain substances in the blood, such as homocysteine and fibrinogen, have been linked to heart disease. There is also some evidence to suggest that a common bacterium that is often responsible for respiratory infections—*Chlamydia pneumoniae*—has been found in some of the plaques of atheroma that block the heart's arteries.

IMPAIRED BLOOD SUPPLY

The muscle in the walls of the heart chambers requires a constant supply of oxygen-rich blood to function efficiently. Any reduction or loss of this supply means that the muscle may malfunction or die. The most common cause of impaired blood supply is coronary artery disease, a major killer in the Western world, not just because of our genetic make-up, but also as a result of lifestyle factors, such as smoking and lack of physical activity, and a cholesterol-rich diet. All these are risk factors for the development of atherosclerosis, in which fatty deposits build up in the walls of the arteries. These deposits can eventually

WEAKENED HEART MUSCLE

The pumping strength of the heart is provided by the muscle in the walls of the chambers. If the muscle becomes weakened for some reason, the heart finds it difficult to pump blood around the body—a situation that may in time lead to heart failure. The condition known as dilated cardio-myopathy has just this effect. The heart muscle becomes weak and then stretches so that the chambers, and in particular the left ventricle, enlarge. High blood pressure can also cause thickening and weakening of the heart muscle, as can some infections and an excessive consumption of alcohol on a regular basis.

birth defects

genetics

LESS COMMON

RHEUMATIC FEVER
1.7 million cases reported annually
The number affected is massively reduced from the 1920s, when about 1 in 10 children suffered from this condition.

BRADYCARDIA (A SLOW HEARTBEAT)
5 to 15 per 100,000
(1 in 6666 to 20,000)

ENDOCARDITIS
6 per 100,000
Occurs most often with preexisting heart disease or infection resulting from dental procedures.

How common is heart disease?
The scale above shows a selection of conditions affecting the heart and circulatory system. The figures are for people living in the United States, unless noted otherwise.

atherosclerosis

rhythm problems

block the flow of blood and lead to chest pain (angina) or even a heart attack. Atherosclerosis can also reduce the blood supply to the limbs, particularly the legs, and contribute to the formation of an abnormal clot (thrombosis), an aortic aneurysm, and, if the blood supply is completely cut off, sometimes even gangrene.

HEART VALVE DEFECTS

A series of one-way valves between the chambers of the heart makes sure that blood flows in one direction only. If these valves become damaged, they can create a disturbance in the natural blood flow. Those usually affected are the valves on the left side of the heart—the mitral and aortic valves. If these become narrowed, they prevent the blood from flowing easily from one chamber to another. Alternatively, they can become leaky so that as a chamber contracts, blood flows backward as well as forward. Although many specific disorders can affect the heart valves, the natural aging process inevitably will lead to a certain degree of valve deterioration in all of us.

ELECTRICAL DISTURBANCES

The heart is controlled by a natural pacemaker and synchronized by an elaborate system of wiring. A malfunction in the system can trigger abnormal heart rhythms (arrhythmias), which may be abnormally slow or abnormally fast. In either case, the amount of blood that the heart pumps is reduced, leading to faintness, blackouts, or even sudden death.

A slow heartbeat usually develops if the heart's natural pacemaker, the sinoatrial node, fails to function properly or if the electrical connection between the chambers of the heart is interrupted. In these situations, doctors can replace the heart's natural electrical system with an artificial pacemaker—an effective cure for either problem. A fast heartbeat occurs when electrical impulses arise from an area other than the natural pacemaker. One particular arrhythmia, atrial fibrillation, is extremely common, particularly in elderly people, and although it sounds dramatic, it does not usually affect day-to-day life and is easily treated with medication. At the other end of the scale, however, is

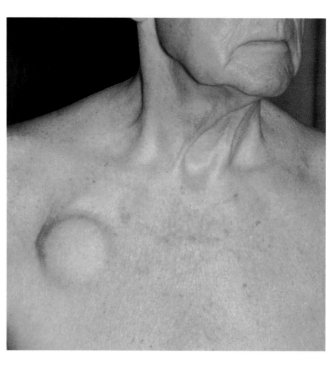

A heart pacemaker
If the heart itself is unable to create sufficient electrical impulses, doctors can insert a pacemaker. This small device is inserted under the skin to supply the missing impulses.

ventricular tachycardia, which can have fatal consequences unless doctors act rapidly.

INFECTION

Rheumatic heart disease following rheumatic fever in childhood was once by far the most common cause of heart valve disease in the Western world. Improvements in housing conditions and the introduction of antibiotics led to a steep decline in cases of rheumatic fever during the 20th century, and rheumatic heart disease is now extremely rare. Nevertheless, other infections, although uncommon, can affect any of the heart's layers.

The membrane that surrounds the heart, the pericardium, can become inflamed and cause sharp chest pain as the heart rubs against it. This type of infection is called pericarditis and is usually caused by a virus. Viral infection can also cause severe, sudden inflammation of the muscle layer of the heart, known as myocarditis. Heart valves that are faulty, or replacement valves, are far more vulnerable to infection than healthy ones. This type of infection—endocarditis—is caused by bacteria traveling in the bloodstream to the valves from another source of infection, such as the teeth.

Recent research has shown that infection with the bacterium *Chlamydia* may contribute to the development of coronary artery disease.

What is a heart murmur?

There are particular sounds heard through the stethoscope that doctors call *heart murmurs*. Blood normally flows "quietly" between the chambers of the heart. But turbulent blood flow creates "noise" as it gushes around the heart; this is what doctors call a murmur. Such murmurs are common, especially among young people, but in some cases a murmur can indicate the existence of a faulty heart valve that is not shutting or opening properly between beats.

ASK THE EXPERT

Recent studies have shown that people of working age are 20 percent more likely to have a heart attack on a Monday compared with the average for other days of the week.

Meet the cardiovascular experts

Doctors, nurses, and technicians work as a team to diagnose and treat heart and circulatory disease. Specialized training and years of experience contribute to the overall care of the thousands of patients who are treated each year in the United States.

CARDIOTHORACIC SURGEON

The cardiothoracic surgeon works closely with the cardiologist and performs a range of complex operations, including restoring blood flow to the heart or replacing faulty or damaged heart valves. Not every hospital has this specialist surgeon.

VASCULAR SURGEON

A vascular surgeon specializes in operating on blood vessels and often treats the same patients as the cardiothoracic surgeon—a patient who has coronary artery disease is also likely to have problems with other arteries. If blockages occur in blood vessels elsewhere in the body, the vascular surgeon can carry out complicated surgical procedures to bypass what may be a life-threatening condition. In particular, a weakened wall in the aorta, known as an aortic aneurysm, is often treated by replacing the damaged section with artificial material. A vascular surgeon would also operate on varicose veins.

CARDIAC TECHNICIAN

The technical side of cardiac investigation relies heavily on cardiac technicians, who take responsibility for the supervision and interpretation of a range of diagnostic tests and procedures. These include electrocardiography (ECG), 24-hour ECG monitoring, and diagnostic ultrasound of the heart, called echocardiography. The cardiac technician is an essential member of the team in the cardiac catheterization laboratory, where responsibilities include monitoring the patient's condition throughout the procedure.

CARDIAC NURSE

Nurses who specialize in diseases of the heart have the expertise required to work in cardiac care units—wards that use high-tech heart-monitoring equipment. They look after and counsel patients and their relatives during and after heart attacks or after heart surgery. Some cardiac nurses are specialists in rehabilitation and run exercise programs, in conjunction with physical therapists, for patients recovering from heart attack or surgery.

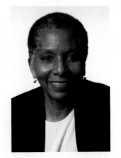

CARDIOLOGIST

A cardiologist is a hospital-based doctor who specializes in diseases of the heart. Not only do cardiologists diagnose heart disease and decide on treatment, but they also undertake a range of invasive and noninvasive procedures. These include cardiac catheterization and coronary angiography, insertion of permanent pacemakers, and echocardiography.

PERFUSIONIST

During some types of cardiac surgery, the patient's heart is deliberately stopped and the job of the heart and lungs is taken over by a heart–lung machine (see page 122). The perfusionist is the technician responsible for maintaining and running this delicate and crucial piece of machinery as well as monitoring the patient's temperature and the levels of oxygen in the blood.

PHYSICAL THERAPIST

Nowadays, patients are encouraged to get up and around as soon as possible following cardiac or vascular surgery, and a previously fit person may be discharged from the hospital within a week. This is where the physiotherapist comes in. Gentle mobilization and breathing exercises, which are started within days of a heart attack or surgery, play an important role in avoiding postoperative complications such as deep vein thrombosis or chest infections. In addition, physical therapists are involved in running long-term rehabilitation programs for patients following a heart attack or surgery.

FINDING OUT WHAT IS WRONG

Doctors have access to a wide range of sophisticated equipment that allows them to look at the heart from every angle, to check whether it is functioning properly, and to monitor its blood supply and electrical activity. In many cases, a simple blood test will provide vital information but more complex investigations are usually required to make a definite diagnosis. In addition to the routine ECG, there are a variety of imaging techniques available that all contribute to the diagnostic picture.

Medical history and examination

Family history, lifestyle, and the sound of the heart beating form the basis on which many diagnoses are made. All this information and more is provided during the initial meeting.

MEDICAL HISTORY—THE FIRST STEP TO DIAGNOSIS

An initial visit to your family doctor with symptoms of possible heart disease may well lead to a referral to a heart specialist—a cardiologist. Like all doctors, cardiologists rely on a description of the symptoms to provide them with a basis on which to build their diagnosis. Although laboratory tests and imaging provide a great deal of information, a symptom such as pain can be described only by the individual concerned. A communicative and open relationship between patient and doctor is therefore vital, and any withheld information could slow the diagnostic process.

General information about symptoms

The doctor will want to hear about the physical symptoms and will also show particular interest in any family history of heart problems, as well as the nature of

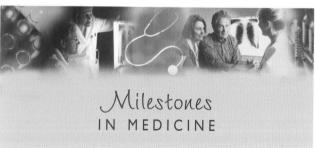

Milestones
IN MEDICINE

The stethoscope was invented by a French physician, Rene Theophile Hyacinthe Laënnec, in 1816 during an examination of one of his female patients. Back then, the usual technique was to feel the heartbeat by placing a hand on the chest, but his patient was too overweight and the physician thought it would be improper to place his ear there. Improvising, he rolled up a piece of paper, placed one end over her heart and the other to his ear, and was amazed by the clarity of the sounds.

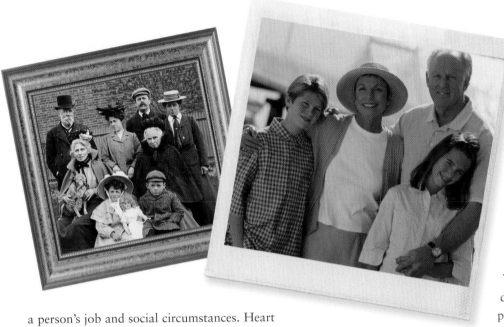

Handed down from generation to generation
Heart disease and high blood pressure in particular tend to run in families, so doctors will quiz you about your family's medical history.

a person's job and social circumstances. Heart disease is inextricably linked to lifestyle—Hardly a week goes by without media coverage of lifestyle risk factors or ways to reduce the incidence of heart conditions. Information about a person's career and lifestyle is therefore essential, not to give doctors ammunition for a lecture, but to enable them to identify risk factors for particular diseases. For example, chest pain in a man over 65, who smokes cigarettes and also eats a high-fat diet, is very likely to be caused by coronary artery disease.

The physical symptoms themselves often give a clear indication of the problem. Particularly important in diagnosing heart disease is whether the symptoms improve or worsen under certain conditions, such as exercise or rest. The cardiologist will also want to know about any previous heart problems, for example a heart attack or bypass operation, or known heart valve disease, which can help in the interpretation of new symptoms.

Symptom specifics

Chest pain is one of the most common symptoms of heart disease and can be a frightening experience, instantly instilling fears of a heart attack into many people. Pain in the chest, though, is not always a sign of heart disease: It could be caused by severe indigestion or inflammation of the muscles of the chest wall. Equally, breathlessness can be a sign of heart failure or angina, but is often a symptom of a lung condition, such as bronchitis, or may simply be caused by a lack of fitness or by being overweight.

The fact that there are many possible diagnoses means that a careful description of each symptom, its severity, how long it lasted, and under what conditions it started

are of great importance— These details will help the doctor most. For example, pain in the chest that worsens when walking up a hill or that travels down the arm may indicate angina, whereas breathlessness when lying flat, or waking up fighting for breath, are both characteristic symptoms of heart failure rather than a problem with the lungs.

Past medical information

A person's medical history is always of great importance to the doctor. New symptoms could mean that an existing medical condition is getting worse or that the treatment is not necessarily working. Heart disease can also develop as a complication of another condition. High blood pressure is a good example of this, as consistently elevated blood pressure can put strain on the heart and eventually contribute to a heart attack. Being aware of the existence of such conditions helps doctors piece together the whole picture and decide on further investigations.

THE PHYSICAL EXAMINATION

Without making a conscious effort, the doctor will have started the physical examination while taking the patient's medical history. Simply looking at the patient is enough to start the process. What is the overall picture—healthy or unwell? Are there any obvious signs of pain? Is the person struggling for breath?

Listening to heart sounds

Almost two centuries after it was first invented, the stethoscope remains one of the most valuable tools for diagnosis. The stethoscope is placed in four different positions on the chest, each of which gives information about a different heart valve. A normal heartbeat consists of a double sound (the characteristic lubb-dupp), which is made by the snapping shut of the valves after the heart chambers have contracted. Cardiologists are able to detect any abnormal or extra sounds that might signify heart disease. For instance, a "heart murmur" is the noise of turbulent blood flow within the heart, which could indicate a diseased valve.

Checking the heart rhythm

Feeling the pulse at the wrist gives the cardiologist a good indication as to the rate, rhythm, and strength of a person's heartbeat. In a healthy adult, the heart rate is between 60 and 80 beats per minute but it can vary depending on a person's level of fitness. A much faster or slower rate than normal, or an obvious irregularity in rhythm, may indicate an abnormality.

Assessing fluid balance

The heart is responsible for pumping blood around the body, and the blood is a vehicle for removing excess water; any problem with the pump can lead to a build-up of fluid. Sometimes, retained water is clearly visible; for example, a person with heart failure may have swollen ankles. If fluid has gathered on the lungs, the doctor is able to hear "crackles" through the stethoscope.

Checking for damaged arteries

One major cause of disease is atherosclerosis in which the arteries in the body become clogged, slowing the blood flow. To check if the blood is flowing freely through the body, the doctor may feel for key pulses.

The body's pulse points
The beating of the heart can be felt at certain points in the circulatory system; inability to hear one could indicate a blockage.

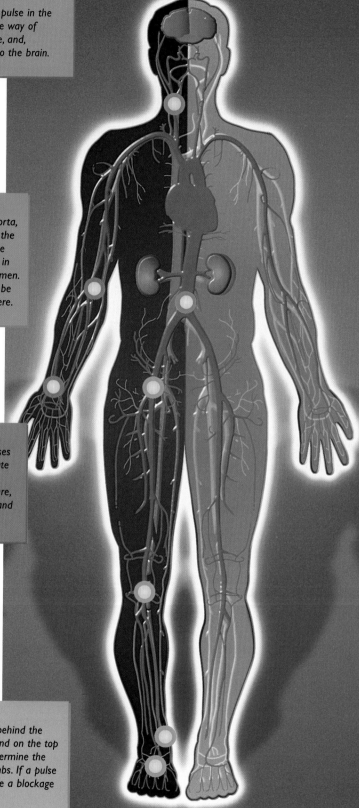

CAROTID PULSE
Feeling and listening to the pulse in the carotid artery is an accurate way of assessing heart rhythm, rate, and, sometimes, the blood flow to the brain.

ABDOMINAL PULSE
The pulsating of the aorta, the main motorway of the arterial network, can be felt only in thin people in the center of the abdomen. Aortic aneurysms may be diagnosed by feeling here.

ARM PULSES
The most common pulses used to assess heart rate and rhythm, and to determine blood pressure, are those at the wrist and the inside of the elbow.

LEG PULSES
These pulses—in the groin, behind the knee, just below the ankle, and on the top of the foot—are used to determine the blood supply to the lower limbs. If a pulse cannot be felt, it may indicate a blockage in one or more arteries.

Measuring blood pressure

A key part of the physical examination is measuring the pressure of the blood within the arteries of the body. A straightforward and revealing observation, blood pressure is an important factor in both the diagnosis and the prevention of heart disease.

What is blood pressure?

Blood pressure refers to the pressure in the arteries, which is measured at two stages—as the heart contracts and pushes blood into the circulation (systolic) and when the chambers of the heart are refilling with blood between beats (diastolic). A blood pressure measurement is expressed in millimeters of mercury as systolic pressure over diastolic pressure.

During an average day, blood pressure constantly changes, depending on many practical factors, such as whether we are moving around or relaxing and even whether we are standing, sitting, or lying down. Primarily, though, blood pressure is controlled by the amount of blood pumped from the heart and the resistance of the walls of the arteries. In a healthy person, the fluctuating pressure remains within an acceptable range and does not create any problems. If blood pressure becomes high, however, and remains so, it may be necessary to begin long-term drug treatment to reduce the risk of heart disease and stroke. As a general guide, doctors will probably show concern if a person consistently has a systolic pressure greater than 140 millimeters of mercury or a diastolic pressure greater than 90 millimeters of mercury.

How is it measured?

The conventional method of measuring blood pressure is with a manual sphygmomanometer. This consists of an inflatable cuff with two tubes—one connected to a hand pump and the other to a pressure gauge containing a column of mercury (see page 48). These are gradually giving way to automatic blood pressure machines, which are accurate as well as very easy to use: The cuff is connected to a machine that at the press of a button inflates the cuff and provides a digital readout of blood pressure and heart rate within seconds. In an intensive care unit, blood pressure is sometimes measured continuously via a cannula—a narrow, hollow tube—placed directly into an artery in the arm.

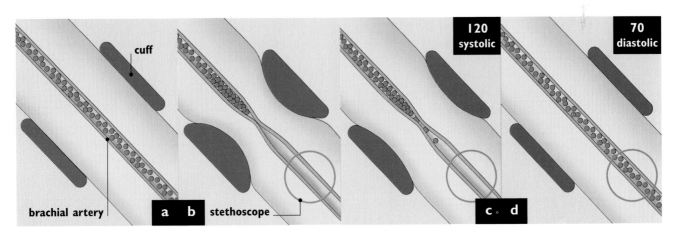

cuff

120 systolic

70 diastolic

brachial artery   **a** **b** **stethoscope**   **c** ∘ **d**

How blood pressure is measured

a An inflatable cuff attached to a pressure gauge is placed around the upper arm so that it is positioned over the main artery—the brachial artery.

b The doctor or nurse inflates the cuff to block the flow of blood through the artery, while placing a stethoscope on the arm just below the level of the cuff, on the inside elbow.

c The cuff is then gradually deflated. The first audible beat indicates the returning blood flow through the artery—this is known as the systolic pressure.

d As the cuff deflates further, there comes a point when the pulse is silent. This occurs as blood begins to flow smoothly again and is called the diastolic blood pressure.

Testing blood samples

Normal levels of the abundant chemicals present in blood were established by scientists many years ago. Any change in a particular level, or the detection of a substance that is not normally present, can provide doctors with a wealth of information.

Blood samples are usually taken from a vein at the inner elbow—a slightly uncomfortable but not usually painful experience. Depending on the tests required, blood samples may end up in different laboratories, so several test tubes are often filled from one sample. Once in the laboratory, levels of chemicals are measured by machines.

DETECTING DAMAGE TO HEART MUSCLE

Damaged heart muscle leaks particular enzymes into the bloodstream almost immediately. A simple blood test to confirm the presence of three of these enzymes—creatine kinase, cardiac troponin I and T (CTRPI; CTRPT), and myoglobin—usually confirms a diagnosis of heart attack. The enzymes rise and fall in a characteristic time pattern so are monitored for at least 24 hours at 8-hour intervals.

Because of recent advances in technology, it is possible to measure specific substances that are released from a damaged heart. The most common of these are troponin I and troponin T, both of which are elements of the contracting system within heart muscle cells. If a patient experiencing chest pain shows low levels of troponins in the blood, it is unlikely that a heart attack is the cause.

CHECKING LIPID LEVELS

There is now firm evidence that high levels of certain fatty substances (lipids) in the blood, particularly cholesterol and triglycerides, are strongly linked to the development of coronary artery disease. More important, experts are certain that in people who already have heart disease, lowering an even modestly raised cholesterol level significantly reduces the risk of further complications. Doctors, therefore, routinely take a blood sample to measure lipids in people with existing or suspected heart disease.

TESTING BLOOD SUGAR LEVELS

People with diabetes mellitus have a greater risk than normal of developing heart disease. If the doctor suspects that a person has heart disease, he or she will probably check the level of sugar in the blood as part of the routine investigations. This type of blood test can be done on the spot by pricking the finger. A drop of blood is placed onto a test stick and inserted into a tiny machine, which provides a digital read-out. If the blood sugar is within normal limits, it is unlikely that a person has diabetes, but if it is elevated, then further tests may be necessary.

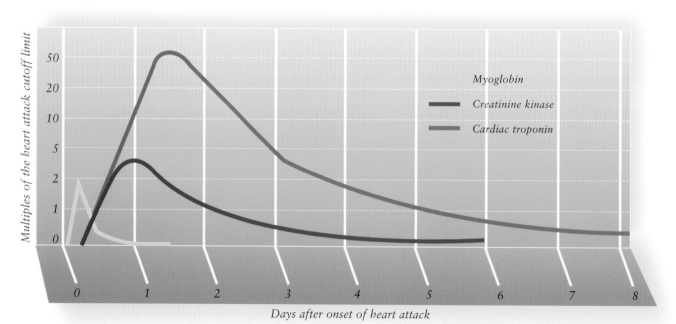

Monitoring the heart's electricity

The heart relies on highly synchronized electrical impulses to function properly. Electrocardiography provides experts with a complete picture of the electrical activity in the heart, so they can analyze the data and detect any faults in the system.

What is it used for?

The heart contains its own electrical signal generator, which can function completely independently from the rest of the body. If something goes wrong, however, there is no back-up, and doctors must act quickly to restore normal function. Often, the difficulty is knowing exactly what is wrong. One of the most revealing investigations, particularly if doctors suspect a heart attack, is the electrocardiogram (ECG). During this procedure, electrodes are placed on the chest and limbs to measure the natural electrical activity of the heart. Changes in ECG readings over time can provide important information about the progress of heart disease.

How does it work?

Although an ECG is a simple procedure, the resulting data are complex and interpretation requires expert knowledge. In its simplest form, three sticky electrodes are placed at specific points on the chest and connected to a heart monitor to give information on screen about the basic heart rate and rhythm. More detailed information can be obtained by doing a 12-lead ECG, so called because it consists of 12 separate tracings, which are all printed out on a single sheet of paper. The procedure takes only a few minutes; the most lengthy part is the application of 10 electrodes (only 10 are required to produce the 12 tracings), 1 on each limb and 6 across the front of the chest in the region of the heart. The electrodes are then connected via cables to the mobile ECG machine, which because of advancing technology is now no bigger than a computer printer.

Having a 12-lead ECG
Ten sticky electrodes are placed at specific points on the body—1 on each limb and 6 on the chest. The electrodes pick up electrical impulses in the heart and relay them to the ECG machine, which produces the tracing.

Reading the result

Each tracing gives an electrical view of the heart from a slightly different angle and comprises a characteristic set of waveforms that indicate different phases in one heartbeat. For example, the so-called "P-wave" is an upward wave that represents the electrical activity as the heart's collecting chambers—the atria—contract and push the blood into the pumping chambers or ventricles. This is followed by the "QRS complex," which indicates the activity as the ventricles contract, pushing the blood into the body's circulation. After a further delay comes the "T-wave," representing the recovery of the ventricles.

Experienced cardiac specialists examining these waveforms can make diagnoses simply by measuring the

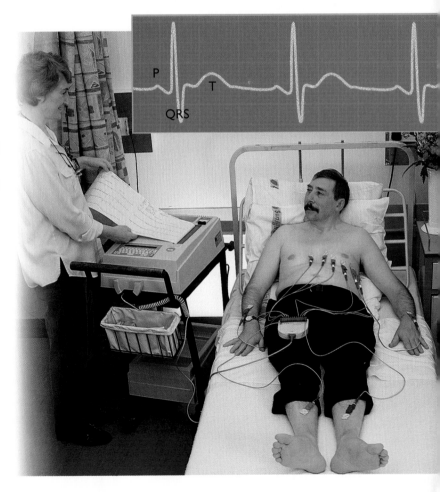

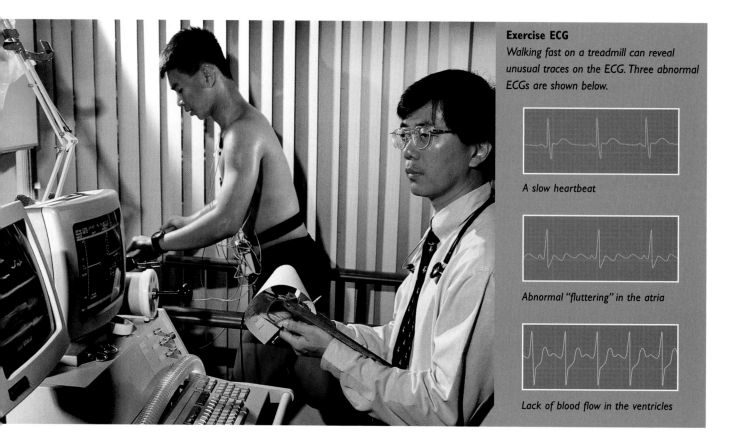

Exercise ECG
Walking fast on a treadmill can reveal unusual traces on the ECG. Three abnormal ECGs are shown below.

A slow heartbeat

Abnormal "fluttering" in the atria

Lack of blood flow in the ventricles

gap between successive QRS complexes and by looking at the general patterns and shapes of the waves. Conditions such as high blood pressure, heart attack, or angina often show distinct abnormalities that are immediately recognizable. Looking at an ECG recorded during an episode of angina can sometimes give a clue as to which area of heart muscle is involved and therefore which coronary artery is blocked.

24-hour ECG recording

One of the difficulties of using ECG to diagnose suspected heart rhythm disturbances is that the abnormality may not actually occur during the procedure. To try to obtain a tracing while a person is experiencing symptoms, doctors sometimes issue a 24-hour ECG recorder, which is no bigger than a personal stereo, so it doesn't interfere with daily life. Sometimes the symptoms may be so infrequent that they cannot even be captured over a 24-hour period, and in such cases an event monitor is often loaned to the patient for a few weeks, or sometimes even longer, and is activated only when symptoms occur.

Modern technology enables rhythm tracings from an event monitor to be transmitted to the hospital by telephone so that a diagnosis can be made.

Exercise ECG testing

Often, standard ECGs are normal in people with angina, as the blood supply to the heart muscle is perfectly adequate at rest. A procedure called exercise ECG testing, as its name implies, combines graded exercise with ECG recording in an attempt to bring on the symptoms of angina. The test provides data about existing heart disease, as well as information about the likelihood of a future heart attack.

The idea of creating an episode of angina is fairly worrying to many people, but the procedure is supervised by two staff members, one of whom is a doctor, and an experienced technician. The most commonly used equipment is a treadmill with a gradual increase in speed and gradient, although some hospitals use an exercise bicycle. The person is monitored throughout the procedure using a 12-lead ECG, and blood pressure is measured during each exercise stage. Exercise continues until either the person becomes tired or experiences chest pain or breathlessness, or the staff supervising the test become concerned about the blood pressure measurements or the heart tracing.

Imaging structure and function

For over a century, doctors have been using X-rays to look inside the body for damage or disease. Today, imaging technology continues to advance and techniques such as echocardiography, MRI, and radionuclide scanning provide minutely detailed images of the heart.

CHEST X–RAY

Despite the range of sophisticated imaging techniques available, a plain X-ray of the chest is often the first step on the diagnostic ladder. It provides a great deal of information about the heart safely, simply, and painlessly, and it is also very good value for the money. However, because a certain amount of radiation is involved, X-rays are not taken if a woman is pregnant because it could harm her unborn baby.

What is it used for?

A plain X-ray provides doctors with a basic but clear view of the heart and lungs. Looking at the shape and size of the heart as a whole is often enough to give an indication of where a problem lies—For example, the diameter of the heart often increases during heart failure. The shape and size of specific heart chambers can also be clearly seen on an X-ray image. In addition to examining the outline of the heart, doctors will also look at the lungs. In some people with severe heart failure, there may be a noticeable accumulation of fluid in the lung tissue.

How does it work?

The standard chest X-ray is taken from the back, but sometimes a side view is taken as well if doctors need to see the heart from more than one angle. The person usually stands during the procedure, with arms raised to move the shoulder blades out of the way. Just before the X-ray is taken, the X-ray technician will ask the person to take a deep breath to expand the lungs and the rib cage. The whole process takes only a few minutes.

An X-ray machine transmits X-rays of a specific length through the chest onto a carefully positioned photographic plate containing film. As the rays pass through the chest, any dense tissue, such as the heart or bone, slows down their progress and casts a shadow on the film, which appears white. Any tissue that allows the X-rays to travel freely through the chest, like the spaces in the lungs, appear black on the X-ray. Consequently, the heart appears as a white silhouette with the dark lungs on either side enclosed in a white rib cage.

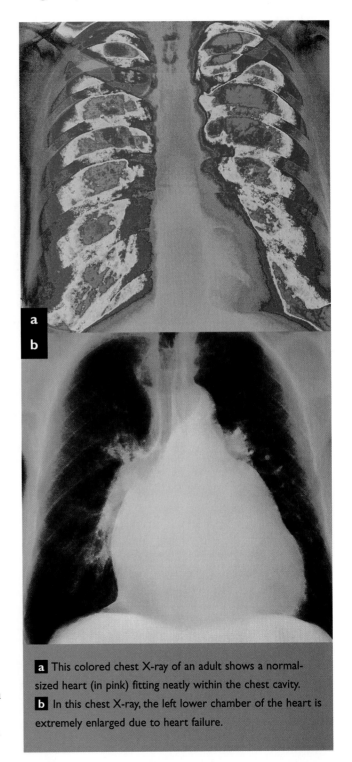

a This colored chest X-ray of an adult shows a normal-sized heart (in pink) fitting neatly within the chest cavity.

b In this chest X-ray, the left lower chamber of the heart is extremely enlarged due to heart failure.

ECHOCARDIOGRAPHY

Ultrasound scanning of the heart, known as echocardiography (echo for short), has revolutionized cardiovascular medicine over the past 20 years. It provides detailed information about the heart's structure and function that was previously available only through invasive techniques such as cardiac catheterization. Echocardiography is entirely safe: It is noninvasive, free from radiation exposure, and can be performed in a clinic or at the hospital bedside. Using simple sound waves, this technique is able to pick out areas of poor blood supply or muscle damage. Until recently, the images created by the scanning procedure—known as echocardiograms—have given doctors only two-dimensional views of the heart, but 3-D applications are now becoming available.

Using echo, doctors can examine the heart of a fetus while in the uterus to detect congenital heart defects.

What is it used for?

Echocardiography allows doctors to visually inspect the heart's valves and chambers, providing information on:
- the overall arrangement of the chambers and valves;
- heart size;
- the heart muscle and how well it is pumping (areas of thinning or loss of contraction in the muscular wall of the left ventricle may indicate a previous heart attack);
- the heart valves and their structure, how blood is flowing across them, and whether there is any backward leakage (regurgitation);
- blood flow within the heart.

How does it work?

An echo machine consists of a hand-held probe connected to a large, but wheelable, processing unit with a screen. The probe contains a device known as a piezo-electric crystal that emits high-frequency sound waves (ultrasound). When placed on the outside of the chest, the probe directs ultrasound waves into the body. Just as the sound of your voice will bounce off the walls of an empty room and return to you as an echo, the waves emitted by the probe are reflected off different tissues within the body and travel back to the crystal as "echoes." Not only does the probe emit ultrasonic waves, but it also detects the returning sound waves: The longer a wave takes to return to it, the farther away the tissue is. The computer processes the information from the probe to build up a black-and-white, 2-D picture of the heart on a screen; this

HAVING AN ECHOCARDIOGRAM

The doctor started by explaining that the procedure was exactly the same as having an ultrasound scan.

I felt more relaxed, then, as it was something that my daughter had described to me after having it done on several occasions during her pregnancies. I was asked to remove my clothes down to my waist and then hop onto the table. The doctor positioned me lying slightly on my left side with my arm behind my head during the procedure. He told me that this was because the heart is enclosed in a bony cage—the rib cage—and it

can only be viewed through the spaces between the ribs from specific positions, called "echo windows."

The doctor spread some jelly over the skin of my chest, then moved a probe back and forth over the area of my heart. If I turned my head slightly, I was able to watch the images on a screen and could actually see and hear my heart beating. The whole

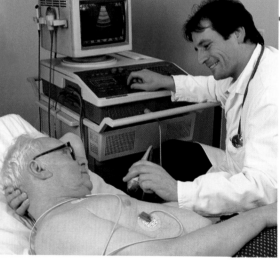

procedure was over in about 15 minutes and the doctor was able to tell me then and there what the problem was.

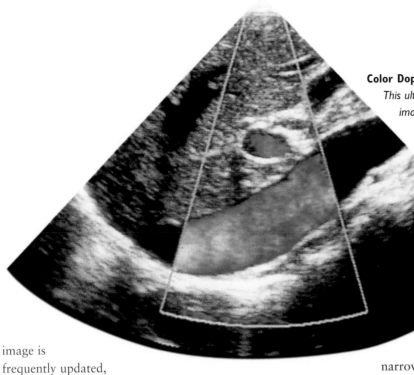

Color Doppler echocardiogram
This ultrasound technique uses sound waves to create an image of the heart and measure the blood flow through the chambers. High-speed blood in one of the heart's arteries is shown in red, and the slower-moving blood in a heart chamber is represented in blue.

image is frequently updated, giving the doctor a moving image of the heart beating in real time.

When ultrasound waves reflect off a moving boundary, such as red blood cells within the heart, the frequency of the returning waves varies, depending on whether the blood cells are moving toward or away from the probe. This phenomenon is known as the Doppler effect, after the physicist who first discovered it—Johann Christiann Doppler. At the flick of a switch, the echo machine can measure not only the speed and direction of blood flow but also color code this movement (usually red for blood moving away from the heart, blue for blood flowing toward the heart) and superimpose this on the 2-D picture (see above).

Stress echocardiography

Not everyone is suited to undergoing an exercise ECG (see page 104), and for these people, doctors skilled in this particular technique may arrange for a "stress echo." For those who are unable to run on a treadmill, the heart is stimulated using a drug. An injection of dobutamine is given to the patient through a vein in the arm, and the dose is gradually stepped up to make the heart muscle beat harder. The basic procedure is the same as with standard echocardiography, but, for safety reasons, the patient is monitored with ECG and blood pressure readings, which are taken at regular intervals. Echo pictures from different viewpoints are recorded before the drug is given and at each dosage increase. The doctor gives the drug and watches the screen for changes as the

drug takes effect. Healthy areas of heart muscle contract harder as the dose of dobutamine increases, but areas supplied by a narrowed coronary artery cannot increase their blood supply adequately and stop contracting.

Transesophageal echocardiography

In some people who are overweight, or women with large breasts, doctors are unable to obtain quality images by echocardiography. In these cases, what is known as a transesophageal echo may be used instead, in which a small probe is passed down the esophagus to provide a view of the heart from inside the body.

AT THE LEADING EDGE

Advancing diagnostic echo techniques

The quality of imaging obtained by echocardiography today is significantly better than that of five years ago. Recent advances in the field include the use of computer processing to take 2-D echo images and assemble them into 3-D reconstructions of the heart. These models will be invaluable to surgeons, who can take a virtual journey in and around the heart and plan their surgical maneuvers in advance. Scientists have also developed special agents that provide previously unheard of levels of detail of the heart and its blood flow. These agents are tiny gas-filled bubbles that reflect ultrasound waves; when injected into the bloodstream, they appear very bright on the image.

RADIONUCLIDE SCANNING

Often termed nuclear cardiology, radionuclide techniques provide an important insight into heart function. This type of imaging is not only invaluable in deciding which patients would benefit from invasive investigations, such as cardiac catheterization or angiography, but may also provide extra information to help in the interpretation of the images obtained during angiography.

What is it used for?

There are several radionuclide techniques, all of which provide an accurate assessment of heart function. The most commonly used techniques are perfusion scanning, which measures the blood supply to the heart muscle, and multiple gated image acquisition analysis (MUGA scan), which assesses the pumping function of the left ventricle. A slightly more sophisticated form of perfusion scanning is single photon emission computed tomography (SPECT). This technique provides a three-dimensional perspective of the heart and can be used to assess heart muscle function and look at blood flow.

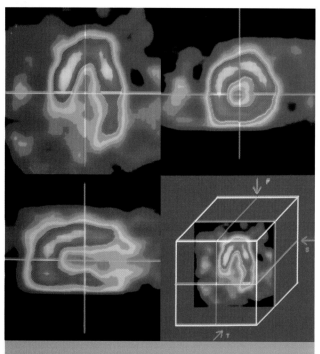

Color SPECT scan

These scans are cross sections of a healthy heart showing blood flow (in red and yellow) to the heart muscle. The last image combines the angles, each indicated by a colored line.

How does it work?

For all the scans, minute amounts of radioactive materials called radionuclides are injected into the bloodstream. These circulate in the blood to and from the heart, emitting a type of radiation known as gamma rays. These rays are detected using a special device called a gamma camera, which can be positioned above and below the patient's body. In MUGA scanning, one view is taken at a time, whereas in SPECT scanning the camera is rotated around the body to create a 3-D picture.

A computer processes the information from the gamma camera and builds up a map of the distribution of the radionuclide within the heart. Doctors then interpret this picture to assess the heart's blood supply and analyze how well the cardiac muscles are contracting.

A perfusion scan enables doctors to visualize the blood supply to the heart muscle. Basically, healthy heart muscle cells absorb the nuclide almost immediately, whereas tissue that has a reduced blood supply absorbs little or none at all. This type of scan can be done both during exercise and at rest, so that doctors can compare the sets of data. Defects that go away at rest represent poor blood supply that is not yet irreversible. Those that remain during rest indicate permanent scarring.

Are there any adverse effects?

These procedures are safe. Although this type of imaging does use radiation, the amount is so tiny, it is lost from the body in a matter of minutes or hours. Because radiation is involved, though, the test is not used on pregnant women or their unborn babies.

MAGNETIC RESONANCE IMAGING (MRI)

MRI produces high-quality images using a powerful magnetic field. The level of detail obtained with MRI is remarkable, enabling doctors to see clearly any abnormalities. MRI can help to define the blood supply to the heart and assess the flow of blood through the heart. It can also provide precise images of the thickness of the heart muscle and the structure of the valves.

The MRI technique uses a powerful magnetic field. The person being scanned lies on a movable bed, which slides inside a large cylindrical magnet. When the magnetic field is switched on, the behavior of the water molecules in the person's body changes, and they produce signals that can be analyzed to produce an image. Although the procedure can appear intimidating, MRI is in fact harmless.

Imaging blood vessels

We have literally thousands of miles of blood vessels in our bodies, any of which can become damaged, blocked, or narrowed. Pinpointing the exact location of an abnormality can be difficult, so tests to image suspect blood vessels are essential diagnostic tools.

DOPPLER STUDIES

A type of ultrasound scanning, Doppler scanning is a safe and accurate technique that is widely used to monitor blood flow through the vessels. By directing high-frequency sound waves from a Doppler probe through the skin to the blood vessels, doctors can obtain vital information about blood flow.

When is it used?

Doppler scanning is used when doctors are concerned that for some reason the arterial blood supply to a particular area of the body is reduced because of a narrowing or a blockage in the blood vessel. This may be caused by atherosclerosis (a condition in which fatty deposits form on the lining of the vessels) or a blood clot. Doppler studies can also be used to detect the presence of a clot in a vein—a deep vein thrombosis.

How does it work?

High-frequency sound waves from the Doppler probe are directed at the affected blood vessels. The probe also picks up and analyzes the "echoes" that return from red blood cells as they travel through the vessels. Amazingly, using this technique, doctors are able to visualize in color the speed and direction of movement of blood through veins and arteries. A system known as Duplex ultrasound uses a similar technique to detect turbulence within the vessels.

ANGIOGRAPHY

Doctors sometimes need to look at the arteries or veins in a certain part of the body or to observe the body's main artery, the aorta. Because blood vessels are hollow and filled with fluid, they do not usually show up on X-rays. In angiography, a radiopaque dye called a contrast medium is injected into the bloodstream before the X-ray is taken, allowing a clear outline of the vessels to be seen.

When is it used?

Angiography is used if doctors suspect a blockage in a blood vessel, caused by a blood clot or atherosclerosis, a condition in which fatty plaques develop on the lining of

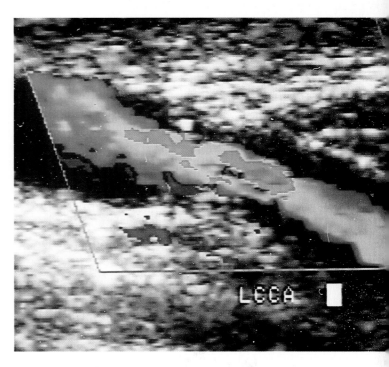

Checking blood flow
A specialized form of ultrasound, Doppler scanning specifically looks at blood flow in vessels and can detect blockages. This scan shows a main artery (yellow and red). The artery visibly narrows in the center because of a build-up of plaques of fatty atheroma, and blood clots (shown in blue) have formed in the narrowed area.

the vessel walls. This technique can also pinpoint the exact location and size of a weakened area of artery, such as an aortic aneurysm, so that appropriate treatment can be prescribed. There are several types of angiography:

- **Peripheral angiography** This is carried out to look at blood supply to the legs and to image the lower aorta.
- **Coronary angiography** During cardiac catheterization, this images the heart's blood supply.
- **Carotid angiography** This checks the carotid arteries, which supply the brain; it is used in certain cases, but Doppler studies are more common as they are safer.
- **Venography** This looks at veins rather than arteries and is usually done to check for deep vein thrombosis.

How does it work?

First, doctors must gain access to the blood circulation through either an artery or a vein. If X-ray images of the arterial blood supply are required, the contrast dye is usually injected via a fine catheter that has been threaded into the circulation through the femoral artery in the groin; sometimes an artery in the arm is used. To look at the venous side of the circulation, the catheter is passed into a vein on the upper side of the foot. A number of X-rays are taken at various stages of the procedure to track the dye through the vessels. Both arteriography and venography are carried out under local anesthetic.

Are there any adverse effects?

The level of radioactivity a person is exposed to during angiography is not hazardous. The main risk following the procedure is bleeding from the puncture site in the groin. To limit the risk of bleeding, a doctor or nurse will apply gentle but firm pressure to the site once the catheter has been removed.

CARDIAC CATHETERIZATION

Each minute the heart pumps an average of 10½ pints of blood around the body. To achieve this, the heart muscle itself demands a healthy supply of oxygenated blood via its coronary arteries. If the supply diminishes,

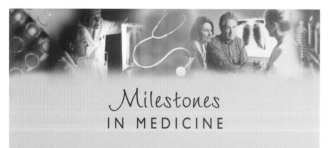

Milestones
IN MEDICINE

In 1929, Werner Forssmann, a German urological surgeon trainee, performed the first human cardiac catheterization—on himself. Using X-ray guidance, he passed a urinary catheter through a vein in his arm all the way into the right side of his heart. Although he eventually won the Nobel prize for his work, at the time the technique was condemned as dangerous, and it was not until the 1960s that the procedure became relatively routine for studying the heart.

not only does the heart muscle suffer, but also the circulation throughout the rest of the body is affected. For more than 50 years, cardiac catheterization has been a common diagnostic technique for looking at the heart muscle's blood supply.

What is it used for?

Cardiac catheterization enables the cardiologist to use angiography (in which dye is injected into blood vessels so they appear opaque on X-rays) to look at the arteries supplying the heart directly, so any blockage or narrowing can be clearly seen. Pressure measurements may be taken throughout the heart to provide information about the efficiency of the pumping mechanisms and the condition of the valves.

How is it done?

Most people nowadays undergo cardiac catheterization as a same-day procedure in a specially designed laboratory. The patient is conscious throughout, but the cardiologist uses a local anesthetic to numb an area of the groin (or occasionally the arm) and then inserts a hollow tube, called a sheath, into the artery beneath. Once this direct access to the arterial side of the circulation is established, a long tube called a catheter is threaded through the groin sheath and, under X-ray guidance, carefully maneuvered up through the blood vessels toward the left side of the heart.

The catheters are specially designed with just the right combination of stiffness and flexibility to allow them to be manipulated. In addition, they have specially shaped tips to help position them in the correct location. First, a "pigtail" catheter is passed into the main pumping chamber of the heart—the left ventricle—and a contrast agent that appears white on X-rays is injected. A moving

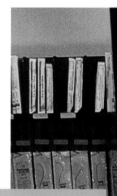

During cardiac catheterization, the patient is lying on his back and is fully awake so he can move slightly if necessary and communicate with the cardiologist. The X-ray machine is positioned close to the body over the area of the heart.

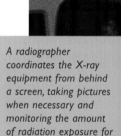

A radiographer coordinates the X-ray equipment from behind a screen, taking pictures when necessary and monitoring the amount of radiation exposure for safety purposes.

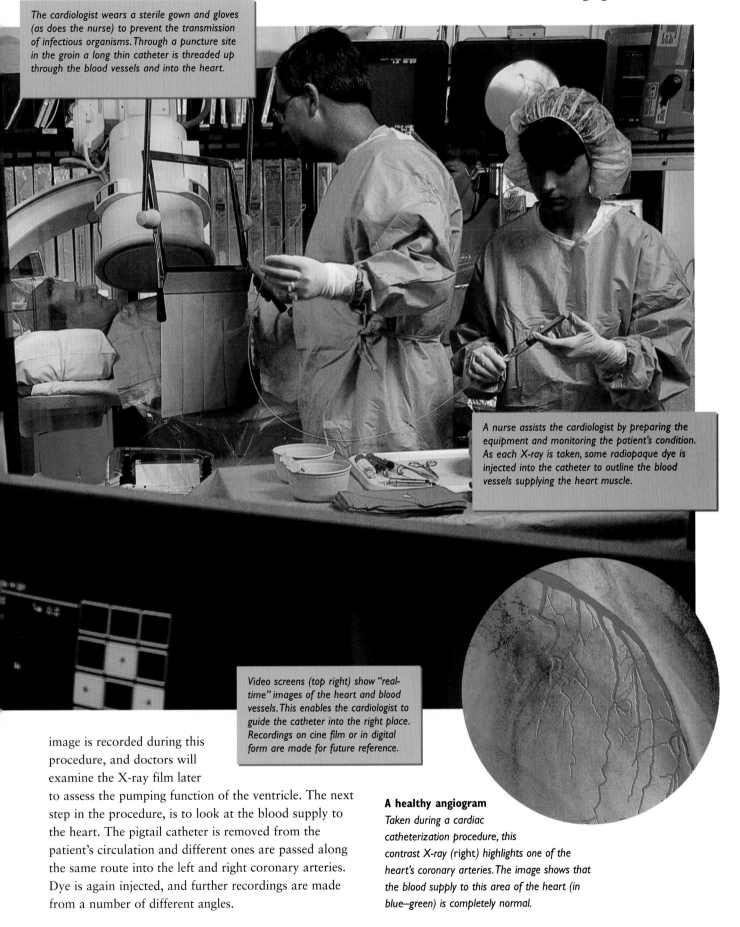

The cardiologist wears a sterile gown and gloves (as does the nurse) to prevent the transmission of infectious organisms. Through a puncture site in the groin a long thin catheter is threaded up through the blood vessels and into the heart.

A nurse assists the cardiologist by preparing the equipment and monitoring the patient's condition. As each X-ray is taken, some radiopaque dye is injected into the catheter to outline the blood vessels supplying the heart muscle.

Video screens (top right) show "real-time" images of the heart and blood vessels. This enables the cardiologist to guide the catheter into the right place. Recordings on cine film or in digital form are made for future reference.

image is recorded during this procedure, and doctors will examine the X-ray film later to assess the pumping function of the ventricle. The next step in the procedure, is to look at the blood supply to the heart. The pigtail catheter is removed from the patient's circulation and different ones are passed along the same route into the left and right coronary arteries. Dye is again injected, and further recordings are made from a number of different angles.

A healthy angiogram
Taken during a cardiac catheterization procedure, this contrast X-ray (right) highlights one of the heart's coronary arteries. The image shows that the blood supply to this area of the heart (in blue–green) is completely normal.

HAVING A CARDIAC CATHETERIZATION

The night before the procedure I wasn't allowed anything to eat or drink after midnight.

In the morning, I arrived at the hospital and was greeted by a nurse who gave me a hospital gown to change into. An intravenous line was put in my arm, and I was given an injection, which made me feel relaxed. Not long afterward I was taken to the cardiac catheterization laboratory.

I moved over onto an X-ray table, and sticky ECG electrodes were attached to my chest. The doctor carefully explained the procedure again to me and then swabbed my right groin with antiseptic and covered the surrounding area with a sterile sheet. She warned me that it might sting when she injected the local anesthetic but that it would only last a few seconds. After that, I felt a slight pushing sensation as the bigger needle and the tube were inserted into the artery in my groin.

When they were ready to take pictures, I was asked to put my arms above my head and hold my breath on and off. During the first injection of dye, I felt a hot flushing sensation passing through my body and was worried that I had passed urine—which of course I hadn't. The doctor did warn me about this, but it still came as a surprise.

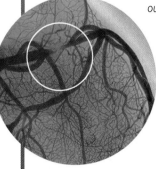

A blocked artery
The white circle marks a severely narrowed or blocked vessel.

After more X-rays, the doctor took out the catheter and pressed on the puncture site for a while to stop the bleeding. Back in the holding area, I lay in bed for a few hours to reduce the risk of bleeding. When my wife came to pick me up, the cardiologist saw us both and explained that they had found a blockage in one of my arteries. At least I didn't have to wait long to hear the results and the recommended treatment.

Sometimes, doctors need to examine the right-hand side of the heart. A second sheath can be inserted into a vein at the groin to provide access to this side. As the catheter is moved through the heart, pressures and blood oxygen levels are measured, while simultaneous recordings are made from the aorta and the left ventricle. Once the doctors have all the information, it is combined to provide a complete picture of the heart's pumping ability and the valves' function.

Are there any risks involved?

Despite the medical staff taking the greatest care, cardiac catheterization is an invasive procedure and sometimes results in a complication. The important thing to remember is that most of these complications are rare. The most common side effect is bruising or bleeding from the groin puncture site; if this happens, a nurse or doctor will apply pressure until the bleeding stops.

In rare cases, the catheter can dislodge a small piece of debris from the wall of the aorta, the largest artery in the body, which could travel to the brain and cause a stroke. Another uncommon complication is the triggering of a heart arrhythmia as the dye is injected into a coronary artery. The tip of a catheter may also damage a coronary artery, causing it to block, particularly if the artery is already severely narrowed. In this event, emergency surgery may be necessary.

New developments in cardiac catheterization

Amazingly, it is now possible to pass a tiny ultrasound probe on the end of a wire to the site of a narrowing in a coronary artery and obtain detailed pictures of the plaque of atheroma—a technique known as intravascular ultrasound. In addition, special wires are now available that actually measure the blood flow down a coronary artery.

CURRENT TREATMENTS

A battery of powerful therapies is currently available to help the heart patient. Dozens of drugs have been developed to control and treat cardiovascular problems, and techniques such as balloon angioplasty can help to avoid the need for surgery. Pacemaker technology is highly advanced, and dramatic surgical procedures to clear and repair arteries, replace valves, and even transplant entire hearts are now almost routine. Rehabilitation services are also available to help the many thousands recovering from heart attacks to resume normal lives and to minimize the chances of further problems.

Drugs for the heart

Heart or circulatory disease can be life-threatening, but, thanks to advances in drug therapy, many conditions can now be successfully controlled without the need for surgical intervention.

DRUGS FOR HIGH BLOOD PRESSURE

An abnormally elevated blood pressure—hypertension—is a strong risk factor for both stroke and coronary artery disease. Drugs to lower blood pressure are, therefore, a vital part of the treatment for hypertension. Sometimes a combination of drugs may be needed. Most drugs have to be taken for more than a month before their effects are evident.

- **Thiazide diuretics** These drugs lower blood pressure by dilating blood vessels and increasing urine output, thereby reducing the amount of water in the bloodstream and the total volume of blood in the circulation. Less blood in the same space means lower pressure. A common example is hydrochlorothezide (also known as HCTZ).

How drugs are administered

Oral Taking drugs by mouth is the most common method. Pills, tablets, and fluids break down in the stomach and the drugs they contain are absorbed through the walls of the intestines. Whether the drug is taken on a full or empty stomach helps to determine the speed and amount of uptake. Check the label instructions to make sure the drug is taken correctly.

Sublingual Tablets are placed under the tongue but not swallowed. They dissolve in the saliva and are quickly absorbed into the bloodstream through the extensive network of blood vessels in the mouth.

Aerosol An inhaler delivers the drug as an aerosol—a cloud of tiny droplets—which is inhaled and reaches the bloodstream through the lungs. Correct technique is important and should be taught to the patient by a qualified practitioner.

Injection Drugs can be rapidly introduced into the body by injecting them. Intravenous administration delivers the drug into the bloodstream as a bolus injection—to a vein—or in diluted form through an intravenous drip. Intramuscular injection delivers the drug to a muscle, usually in the buttock or thigh. Subcutaneous injection delivers a drug just under the skin.

Patches An adhesive patch, impregnated with the drug, is attached to the skin to give a slow-release effect. The drug passes slowly through the skin, eventually reaching the blood.

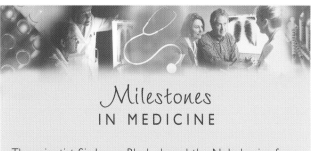

Milestones
IN MEDICINE

The scientist Sir James Black shared the Nobel prize for medicine and physiology in 1988 for his role in the discovery of beta-blockers. These are a much-used and very effective drug treatment for high blood pressure (hypertension) and some heart conditions, such as angina, heart rhythm disturbances, and heart failure. The benefits of beta-blockers are experienced by millions of people throughout the world today.

- **Beta-blockers** These block the effects of epinephrine on the heart and the arteries, slowing the heart rate and relaxing the main arteries to reduce blood pressure.
- **Calcium-channel blockers** These prevent movement of calcium into muscle cells, blocking the contraction of the muscle within the artery wall. With the arteries in a relaxed state there is a fall in blood pressure. Common examples are nifedipine and diltiazem.
- **Angiotensin converting enzyme (ACE) inhibitors** These drugs prevent the production of angiotensin converting enzyme, which is involved in narrowing arteries. They include captopril and enalapril.
- **Angiotensin II receptor antagonists** These are sometimes prescribed if the side effects of ACE inhibitors are too great. They block receptors for angiotensin, preventing it from triggering narrowing of the arteries.
- **Methyldopa** This is most often used for treating high blood pressure in pregnancy, because it is known to be safe for the fetus.

What are the adverse effects?
If you are taking beta-blockers, you may experience cold extremities, tiredness, and impotence. Beta-blockers should not be prescribed to patients with asthma; they can exacerbate the condition. Calcium-channel blockers can cause flushing and headache and are occasionally associated with fluid retention, such as ankle swelling. ACE inhibitors can cause a dry cough, which if persistent can indicate the need for a change in medication.

DRUGS TO LOWER LIPID LEVELS
Abnormally high levels of lipids—cholesterol and triglycerides—in the blood are a major risk factor for the development of atherosclerosis, in which fatty plaques develop inside blood vessels and disrupt blood flow. Lowering high lipid levels using drugs can significantly reduce the risk of heart attacks caused by atherosclerosis.

Cholesterol is essential for many of your body processes and is carried around the body in "containers" called lipoproteins. Two of these lipoproteins—low-density lipoprotein (LDL) and high-density lipoprotein (HDL)—are particularly important for the health of your heart. LDL contributes to the development of atherosclerosis, whereas HDL collects cholesterol from around the body and takes it to the liver for disposal. If changes in diet have proved ineffective at lowering cholesterol levels, the doctor may well prescribe lipid-lowering drugs.

How do they work?
Lipid-lowering drugs work by reducing LDL levels in the bloodstream or by increasing HDL levels so that more lipid than usual is excreted.

Cholesterol and the bile cycle
The liver converts some LDL cholesterol into bile salts, which are released into the intestines to help digest fats. The bile salts, heavy with LDL, are reabsorbed by the small intestine and returned to the liver and broken down, releasing cholesterol back into the bloodstream. Anion-exchange resins disrupt this process.

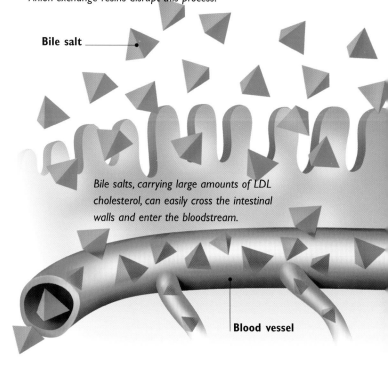

Bile salt

Bile salts, carrying large amounts of LDL cholesterol, can easily cross the intestinal walls and enter the bloodstream.

Blood vessel

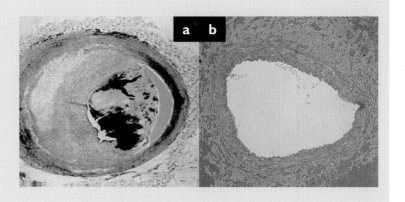

The effects of lipids on your arteries

a The walls of this artery are lined with thick deposits of fatty plaque. The result is a dangerous atheroma, a telltale sign of atherosclerosis, which dramatically reduces the diameter of the vessel.
b Drug treatment can lower overall levels of lipid in the blood and improve the ratio of HDL to LDL cholesterol in the blood, helping to keep arteries clear and unrestricted, as shown here.

- **Statins** These are the most widely used drugs for people at risk of heart disease. By regulating cholesterol production in the liver they reduce total and LDL cholesterol levels in the bloodstream.
- **Fibrates** Another group of drugs known to be effective in lowering lipids. Fibrates are most effective at lowering triglyceride but also reduce LDL and raise HDL cholesterol. These drugs, which include clofibrate and gemfibrozil, are used more frequently when triglycerides only are raised.

- **Anion-exchange resins** These chemicals bind to the cholesterol-carrying bile salts and prevent them from being absorbed in the small intestine. The most commonly used resin is cholestyramine.

What are the adverse effects?

Most lipid-lowering drugs, especially anion-exchange resins, sometimes cause gastrointestinal symptoms, such as constipation, diarrhea, nausea, and vomiting. Rarely, statins can cause a slight abnormality in liver function or muscle weakness.

DRUGS THAT PREVENT BLOOD CLOTTING

Doctors may need to reduce the natural capacity of the blood to clot in certain conditions. For example, if an artery supplying the heart muscle becomes narrowed by fatty plaques, known as atheroma, there is an increased risk of clot formation in that area. This in turn could contribute to further blockage of the artery and a reduction in blood flow to the area of heart muscle, ultimately leading to a heart attack.

Drugs that reduce the clotting potential of the blood, known as anticoagulants, are usually given to protect against heart attack in someone at risk or to prevent further attacks from occurring. These drugs are also used to treat people who suffer from atrial fibrillation or who have replacement heart valves. Such people have a higher risk of a clot forming in the heart, which could predispose them to stroke if the clot blocks an artery in the brain.

How do they work?

There are two main groups: Those that act on the tiny blood cells called platelets that stick together to form the basis of a clot (antiplatelet drugs) and those that interfere with the enzymes and chemical factors in the blood involved in the clotting process (anticoagulants).

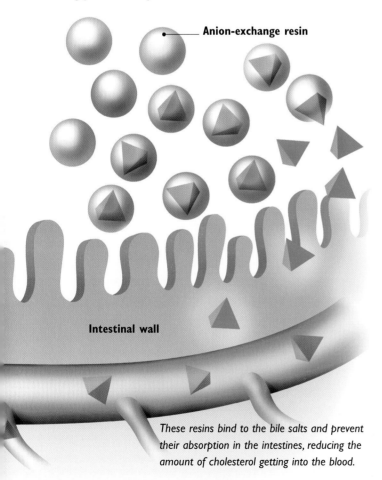

Anion-exchange resin

Intestinal wall

These resins bind to the bile salts and prevent their absorption in the intestines, reducing the amount of cholesterol getting into the blood.

How antiplatelet drugs work

a In normal clot formation, platelets (the small green disks) change shape, becoming spherical, spiky, and sticky, so that they clump together with each other and with red blood cells (large red disks) and strands of fibrin to form clots.

b The micrograph shows a real clot, made up of red blood cells, tiny platelets (only a few are visible), and a white blood cell, all bound up with strands of sticky fibrin.

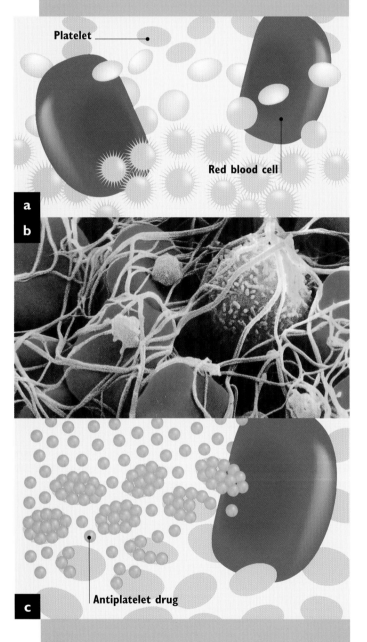

Platelet

Red blood cell

a
b

Antiplatelet drug

c

c Antiplatelet drugs (the tiny orange spheres) prevent clotting by binding to the platelets and stopping them from changing shape or sticking together.

- **Aspirin** This antiplatelet drug reduces the activation of platelets by blocking an enzyme within the cells.
- **Clopidogrel** This fairly new antiplatelet drug is known to be as effective as aspirin in reducing clot formation and is less likely to cause side effects.
- **Coumadin** This is a more potent anticoagulant that blocks the effect of vitamin K, one of the vital factors in the clotting process.

What are the adverse effects?

Aspirin has very few side effects. Some people experience gastric upset, but these symptoms can often be overcome by taking the drug after a meal or with stomach-protecting drugs. People who already have stomach ulcers should avoid aspirin.

Coumadin is associated with an increased risk of bleeding. Every patient responds differently to coumadin, so its effects are closely monitored. It can interact with other drugs; a doctor or pharmacist should always be consulted on any new medication.

DRUGS FOR ANGINA

Angina is the pain caused when the heart muscle is deprived of oxygenated blood, usually due to narrowing of the arteries by atherosclerosis. Drugs for angina can be taken on a regular basis to prevent attacks from occurring and are also available in rapid-action formulas for acute attacks. They are usually taken in pill form but also come as patches, sprays, or sublingual tablets.

How do they work?

There are three groups of drugs used to treat angina, some of which are the same as those used in the treatment of high blood pressure.

- **Nitrates** These dilate the coronary arteries, improving blood flow. The oldest and still most commonly used nitrate, nitroglycerin (NTG), is most effective as a spray or sublingual tablet. Nitrates are also available in longer-acting preparations.
- **Beta-blockers** These cause the heart to beat more slowly by blocking the effects of epinephrine. This in turn reduces the requirement for oxygenated blood so that angina is less likely to develop. Metoprolol and atenolol are commonly used beta-blockers.
- **Calcium-channel blockers** The most commonly used calcium antagonists are nifedipine and diltiazem, both of which work in a similar fashion to nitrates.

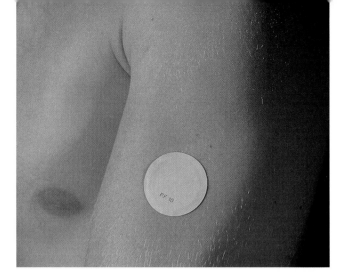

Sticky drugs
Applying a patch containing a particular drug is an efficient way of ensuring a slow and steady dose as it is absorbed through the skin. A person with angina can use nitrate patches to prevent chest pain.

What are the adverse effects?

Nitrates dilate arteries in the head, which can cause flushing and headaches. Vasodilation can also lead to a fall in blood pressure, causing faintness.

DRUGS FOR HEART RHYTHM PROBLEMS

Abnormal heart rhythm problems (arrhythmias) occur when there is a fault in the heart's electrical activity, which sparks the contractions of the heart's pumping chambers (the atria and ventricles). Drugs are frequently used to help return the heartbeat to a normal rhythm.

How do they work?

The choice of drug is dictated by the specific type of heart rhythm disturbance and the underlying cause. Depending on the severity of the condition, the drugs will be given either orally or intravenously in the hospital.

- Beta-blockers These drugs are useful for correcting very fast heart rates such as supraventricular tachycardia. They work by blocking the effect of chemicals that increase the heart rate. The most commonly used beta-blocker is atenolol.
- Calcium-channel blockers Drugs such as verapamil can be used to slow down a rapid heart rate by blocking the flow of calcium into the heart muscle.
- Digoxin This drug is used to treat atrial fibrillation, an abnormal heart rhythm that is particularly common among the elderly. In atrial fibrillation, the heart beats in an

irregular fashion and at a much faster rate than usual (tachycardia). Digoxin works by increasing the strength of the heartbeat and slowing its rate.

- Other drugs If an arrhythmia is more serious—for example, a ventricular tachycardia following a heart attack—more specialized drugs, such as amiodarone, may be prescribed. Coumadin may be prescribed to treat atrial fibrillation, as there is an increased risk of stroke with this particular arrhythmia.

What are the adverse effects?

Many drugs for arrhythmia also lower blood pressure, so a common side effect is dizziness, particularly when standing up from a sitting or lying position. Beta-blockers can result in cold extremities and impotence. Flushing, headache, and swollen ankles have all been experienced by some people taking calcium-channel blockers. Digoxin can cause nausea, vomiting, and diarrhea if the levels exceed certain limits. Amiodarone should only be prescribed under specialist medical supervision, as it can affect lung and liver function and can also result in heightened sensitivity to sunlight. Coumadin affects blood clotting and can increase the tendency to bleed.

DRUGS FOR HEART FAILURE

Any disease that affects the efficiency of the heart can cause heart failure, when the heart is unable to pump enough blood to supply the body's needs. One of the primary features of heart failure is an accumulation of fluid in the circulation, which results in swelling in the body's tissues, particularly the ankles, and shortness of breath brought on by the accumulation of fluid on the lungs. Drug therapy aims to reduce the symptoms of fluid retention and to improve the heart's efficiency.

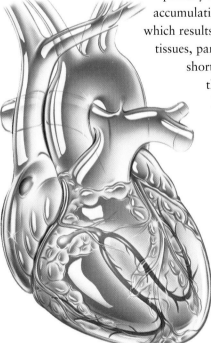

Antiarrhythmic drugs
Different drugs act on different parts of the heart's conduction system to block or slow the passage of electrical impulses. Beta-blockers, for instance, act on the sinoatrial node (green), while digoxin acts on the atrioventricular node (orange).

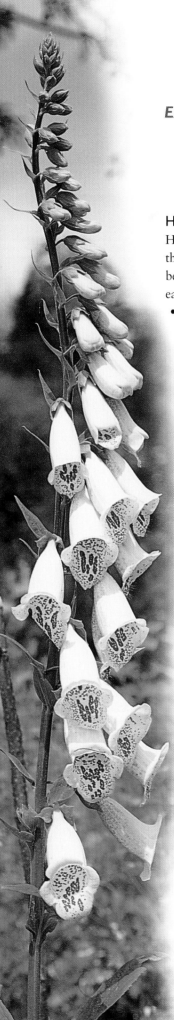

Extract of foxglove—the natural form of digoxin—was found to be effective in treating "dropsy," now known as heart failure, as early as the 18th century.

How do they work?

Heart failure is treated with many of the same drugs as hypertension, partly because relieving high blood pressure eases the workload of the heart.

- **Diuretics** A drug such as furosemide (LASIX) is the mainstay of heart failure treatment. Diuretics cause the kidneys to excrete more sodium and therefore water. The results of a dose of furosemide given intravenously can be spectacular and life saving, particularly in treating fluid on the lungs.
- **Angiotensin converting enzyme (ACE) inhibitors** The vasodilatory effect of these drugs reduces the force needed to pump blood around the body. A commonly used example is captopril.
- **Beta-blockers** Drugs such as metoprolol and atenolol slow down the heart, reducing its workload.
- **Digoxin** This drug is effective in treating heart failure because it helps heart muscle to pump more strongly. It is particularly useful if heart failure is also causing an arrhythmia such as atrial fibrillation.

What are the adverse effects?

Diuretics are generally safe drugs, but the abrupt urge to pass urine caused by frusemide can be very distressing and may cause incontinence, particularly in the elderly. Long-term use can cause imbalance in the minerals in the blood, which can be serious if undetected. Patients taking diuretics should have a blood test at least once a year—more frequently to begin with. High doses of digoxin are toxic and can cause nausea, vomiting, and diarrhea.

DRUGS FOR DISSOLVING CLOTS

The principal cause of a heart attack is a clot (thrombus) blocking one of the coronary arteries that supplies the heart muscle with oxygenated blood. A thrombus is generally caused by the presence of an atheroma—a mass of abnormal fatty deposits on the lining of an artery. If the area of heart muscle supplied by the artery is starved of blood, it becomes irreversibly damaged. Over recent years, as experts gain an increased understanding of the cause of heart attacks, drugs that can dissolve a thrombus and unblock an obstructed artery have been developed.

How do they work?

The drugs are known as thrombolytic or "clot-busting" drugs and have been shown in numerous studies to improve the outlook of patients if given very quickly after a heart attack. Thrombolytics are given intravenously.

- **Streptokinase** This drug is derived from an enzyme produced by the *Streptococcus* bacterium. Because the body recognizes it as a bacterial toxin, immunity develops to it after one dose, meaning that it cannot be given a second time. Streptokinase works by increasing levels of the enzyme plasmin, which breaks down fibrin—an essential substance in clot formation.
- **Alteplase** This is a synthetically produced drug that works in the same way as streptokinase.

What are the adverse effects?

The main problem with thrombolytics is that for as long as they remain in the bloodstream there is a risk of bleeding. Thrombolytic therapy is therefore not given to patients who have experienced serious trauma or recently undergone surgery, or those who have a history of stomach ulcers or brain hemorrhage.

Unblocking blood vessels

With thousands of miles of blood vessels in the body, it is hardly surprising that blockages occasionally occur. Where possible, it is usually better to resolve the problem using one of a number of procedures that avoid the need for surgery.

BALLOON ANGIOPLASTY

Disease of the arteries is usually caused by a gradual build-up of fatty material, known as atheroma, on the blood vessel walls. In time an artery may become so narrow that it can no longer deliver enough oxygen-containing blood to the tissues. Most commonly, these blockages develop in the arteries supplying the heart muscle and the legs. These narrowings can be resolved using a procedure called angioplasty, in which a tiny balloon is inflated in the narrowed area to stretch it. Although complex, balloon angioplasty avoids the need for surgery and a general anesthetic.

Angioplasty versus surgery

Balloon angioplasty is generally carried out if a patient with a narrowing in a coronary artery is experiencing chest pain on a regular basis, and drug treatment is no longer effective. Angioplasty may also benefit someone with peripheral vascular disease, in which the arteries supplying the legs are so narrowed that the muscles are starved of oxygen, causing severe pain on walking—a symptom known as intermittent claudication.

Rate of inflation

Under local anesthetic, a fine catheter with a small deflated balloon at its tip is inserted into an artery via a puncture hole in the skin, either in the groin or in the arm, and is passed along the vessel until it reaches the narrowed part. The balloon is then gently inflated, compressing the tissue responsible for the blockage and widening the affected area of the artery.

The heart of the matter

If the procedure is used to treat the arteries supplying the heart muscle, it is called coronary angioplasty. It is often performed as part of cardiac catheterization, during which doctors carry out contrast X-rays and pressure readings. If coronary angioplasty does not successfully clear the narrowed artery, the next step is to plan coronary artery bypass surgery for a later date.

About one in three arteries treated with angioplasty will narrow again within four to six months. Doctors can try to prevent this with devices called "stents." A coronary stent is a tiny metal tube that is introduced into the coronary artery just after the balloon catheter and positioned at the site of the narrowing. When the balloon is inflated, the stent expands to press against the inner walls of the artery. Once the balloon has been deflated and removed, the stent remains in place on a permanent basis to hold the artery open, improving blood flow and

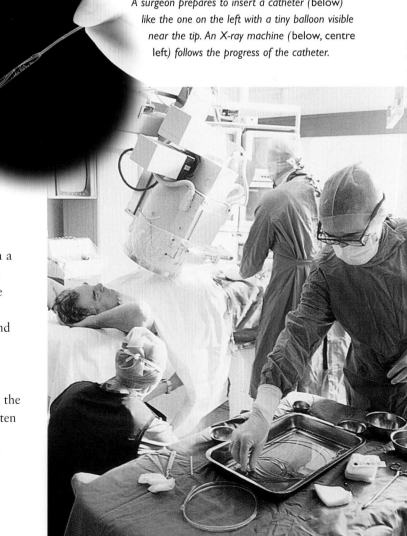

Angioplasty balloon device
A surgeon prepares to insert a catheter (below) like the one on the left with a tiny balloon visible near the tip. An X-ray machine (below, centre left) follows the progress of the catheter.

EXPERIENCING AN ANGIOPLASTY OF THE LEG

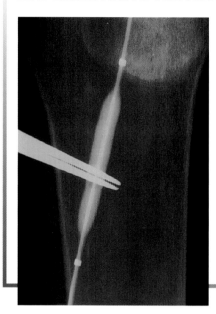

After X-rays and tests, and nothing to eat or drink for hours, the doctor explained what he was going to do.

The worst part was probably getting the local anesthetic, which the doctor injected into my groin, but soon the area was numb. I didn't watch as a sheath and guide catheter were inserted and moved into place. The doctor followed their progress with the help of a large X-ray machine pointed at my leg, and injected a dye to improve the image.

Eventually, the balloon catheter was introduced. I watched on the screen as the doctor inflated it in the constricted area. There was a sharp pain in my leg, which faded as the balloon deflated. The doctor repeated the process a few times, then removed the balloon and checked to see that the blood flow through my newly widened femoral artery had improved. The guide catheter was taken out after about 30 minutes, but they left the sheath in for a couple of hours.

relieving the symptoms of coronary artery disease. Stents are expensive, but improved versions used in conjunction with more advanced anticlotting drugs should make the procedure more popular.

A risky business?
Most coronary angioplasty carries little risk: about 96 percent of angioplasty patients experience no serious complications. In some cases, however, the procedure can cause the artery to block up completely, which then requires emergency surgery.

LASER ANGIOPLASTY
For some people, balloon angioplasty does not work, even with a stent in position. One new technology that has been tried in these situations is laser angioplasty, carried out during cardiac catheterization. Laser technology has been used for tissue vaporization and surgery almost since its invention in 1959. The evolution of fiberoptics paved the way to the development of catheters that could be used to transmit the intense light needed for coronary laser angioplasty. Laser catheter systems have been investigated in the reopening of severely blocked coronary arteries, but they have yet to be proven, and many experts have tried and abandoned laser techniques. In general, the approach is not widely used.

CORONARY ATHERECTOMY
If all else fails, doctors may try another new technique called coronary atherectomy. This is performed by different methods, but basically it involves chopping or grinding away part of the offending plaque in the coronary artery using a catheter with a cutting end. It has been shown to be successful in some cases of complex coronary disease. Less is known, however, about its long-term outcome, and the problem of the recurrent narrowing still remains a major limitation.

Light at the end of the tunnel?

Sometimes, the coronary arteries are so badly blocked that it is impossible to find a healthy area on which a graft can be connected to bypass the blockage. A still experimental technique called transmyocardial laser revascularisation offers promise to these patients. A laser is used to create tiny tunnels in the wall of the heart so that blood from within the chambers can directly enter the tunnels to nourish the heart and relieve angina.

Inserting a pacemaker

When the heart's natural electrical system fails, it is possible for doctors to place an artificial "generator," known as a pacemaker, under the skin of the chest. The pacemaker sits fairly close to the heart and fires off electrical impulses when needed.

All hearts have a natural pacemaker—a group of specialized cells that trigger the electrical impulses that run through the entire heart muscle. These impulses cause the muscle to contract, squeezing the chambers of the heart to pump blood around the body. Sometimes, this natural pacemaker or the electrical conduction pathways within the heart fail to function properly, leading to an abnormal heart rhythm, such as a very slow heartbeat—a condition known as bradycardia. In these cases, a replacement pacemaker that can mimic the natural one is often necessary. A battery-powered, electronic device consisting of a generator and electrical leads can supply electrical impulses either at a set rate or on demand.

Implanting the device

Under local anesthetic, an electrode lead is inserted into a vein at the shoulder or the base of the neck. The cardiologist then guides the lead into the correct chamber of the heart using an X-ray screen. The electrode lead is connected to the pacemaker, which is then fitted into a small "pocket" of flesh that the doctor creates between the skin and the chest muscles (it can be easily felt just beneath the skin). The whole procedure takes about 30 to 60 minutes, and may involve an overnight hospital stay. Modern pacemakers are so small that they are almost completely hidden by overlying tissue—a slight swelling may be all that is visible.

Internal shock waves

Some patients with life-threatening disturbances of heart rhythm may need a device called an implantable cardioverter defibrillator to regulate a normal heart rhythm. A modern defibrillator is smaller than a pack of playing cards and is connected to the interior of the heart by a wire passed through a vein. When this device detects a severe abnormality, it delivers a burst of electrical impulses or an electrical shock to restore a normal rhythm. There are two stages to implanting this device; both the electrodes and the defibrillator need to be placed in position. Alternatively, the procedure may be

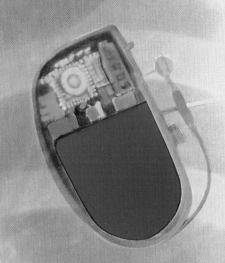

A pacemaker in position
This X-ray clearly shows the pacemaker and electrode wires in position and indicates just how small it is—Modern pacemakers weigh between 2 ounces and 4 ounces. Pacemakers are not affected by X-ray radiation, but some electrical and magnetic equipment can interfere with their operation (see below).

performed by a surgeon working through an open incision in the chest who places large electrodes directly on the outer surface of the heart. If an open operation method has been used, recovery is slower. An open operation is rarely used today.

Life afterward

A person with a pacemaker usually leads a normal life but, because the device is battery powered, the batteries need changing every five to seven years or so. This is a minor procedure that is carried out under local anesthetic.

Some types of electrical equipment can affect pacemakers. Patients should avoid MRI scanners and spot-welding machines, keep mobile phones at least six inches from the pacemaker, and advise airport officials when approaching a metal detector or screening system.

Surgical solutions for heart problems

Nowadays, most heart surgery is routine and safer than ever, thanks to advances in medical technology and surgical equipment. Even though the prospect of heart surgery can be stressful, for many people it offers a welcome resolution to long-term symptoms.

BEFORE SURGERY

Heart surgery can provide welcome relief from a restricted lifestyle, but having an operation is always a worry. Discussing any anxieties with the medical staff and doctors can help to alleviate apprehensions.

Preparing for the operation

Most people are admitted to hospital the day before the operation, unless they are particularly unwell and already an inpatient. Routine blood tests, an electrocardiogram, and a chest X-ray will all be done, and the medical team, comprising doctors, nurses and therapists, will carry out examinations and observations. Patients also need to shave off any excess body hair. For coronary artery bypass grafting, both legs, the groin, and the chest need to be shaved; other types of surgery don't normally require leg shaving. On the day of the operation, a period of "starvation" is necessary beforehand to ensure that the stomach is empty.

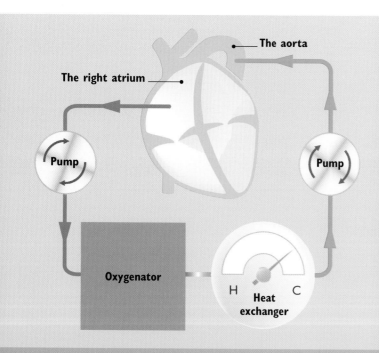

Heart–lung bypass machine

This diagram shows how the circulation is diverted from its normal route. Instead of being sent to the lungs, deoxygenated blood is rerouted from the right atrium through a pump to the oxygenator, where it picks up oxygen. Oxygenated blood then passes through a heat exchanger, which controls its temperature. Another pump drives it into the aorta, from which it can circulate through the body, missing most of the heart.

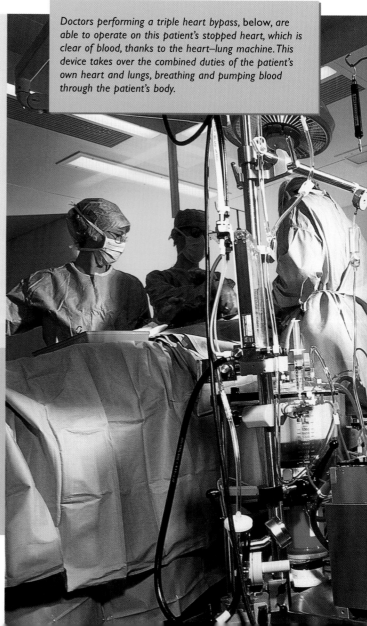

Doctors performing a triple heart bypass, below, are able to operate on this patient's stopped heart, which is clear of blood, thanks to the heart–lung machine. This device takes over the combined duties of the patient's own heart and lungs, breathing and pumping blood through the patient's body.

Postoperative rehabilitation is particularly important in cardiac surgery, so physical therapists and nurses skilled in this specialty usually assess patients before the operation.

Even though this preparation period is a very busy 24 hours, it is also a good time for asking important questions about all aspects of the surgery.

This detail of the heart–lung machine shows blood from the patient's body collecting in the oxygenator. From here it passes through the tubes that make up the heat exchanger (bottom foreground) and then back into the patient's body.

Just before surgery

A premedication injection is given to relax the patient in readiness for the anesthetic. Depending on the operation, a number of monitoring devices will be connected to the patient's body before starting the surgical procedure. Many of these will be put in place by doctors after the anesthetic has taken effect. A fine tube may be inserted into the artery in the arm to measure blood pressure continuously. Other tubes are placed into veins in the arms and neck to enable doctors to give fluid, blood, and drugs to the patient, feeding them directly into the circulation.

TOOLS OF THE TRADE

Every type of surgery lays claim to a selection of specialist equipment, and cardiovascular surgery is no exception. Surgeons use an array of instruments and can call on a range of advanced medical technology. The heart–lung bypass machine is a particularly important piece of equipment used in most types of open heart surgery.

Revealing the heart

With few exceptions, heart operations are performed by cutting through the breastbone. Once an incision has been made vertically down the center of the chest and any bleeding vessels have been closed off, the surgeon divides the breastbone, or sternum, in order to reach the heart. This is done using an electric or compressed air sternal saw, which safely and efficiently splices the sternum in two. The two halves are then eased apart with retractors to reveal the heart. At the close of the operation, the sternum is joined using wire sutures and bone wax that smooths over tiny splinters of bone.

continued on page 126

A perfusionist monitors the heart–lung bypass machine, using it initially to cool the patient's blood, thereby helping to preserve the tissues of the patient's body. Once the surgeons are finished and ready to disconnect the machine at the end of the operation, the perfusionist sets it to reheat the blood gradually returning it to the patient's body temperature.

Heart bypass surgery

First performed in 1967, the coronary artery bypass graft— better known as a heart bypass—is the most common and successful heart operation, prolonging life and restoring vitality to almost one million people worldwide every year.

Coronary artery bypass grafting is now one of the most frequently performed surgical procedures in the United States. The surgery restores the blood supply to damaged heart muscle by providing a new route around one or more blockages in the coronary arteries. Each bypass operation is highly individual, and most take between three and five hours. On average, a patient can expect to stay in the hospital for between five and seven days, with one to four spent recovering in intensive care. The operation has a high success rate, providing immediate and lasting relief from angina for about 8 out of 10 patients who undergo surgery.

The surgical team

A cardiothoracic surgeon performs the delicate maneuvers required to position the bypass grafts on the heart and is assisted by other surgeons on the team. Throughout the operation, an anesthetist administers the general anesthesia, then monitors the patient's heart rate and breathing, while a perfusionist controls the heart–lung machine.

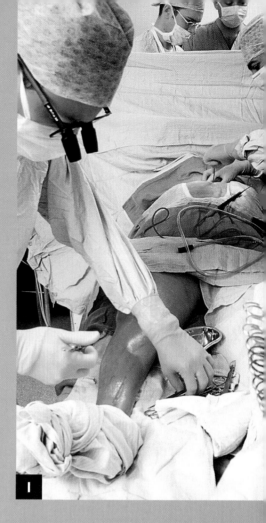

1

A *circuitous route*

Coronary artery bypass grafting involves taking segments of vein from elsewhere in the body to "bypass" the narrowed sections of the coronary arteries and reroute the blood.

The surgeon uses either the internal thoracic artery in the chest or the long saphenous vein from the leg to make the graft. The internal thoracic technique (top) involves redirecting an artery from the chest wall; this technique is suitable for a single graft only.

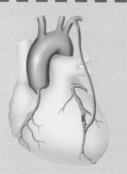

Single bypass *with internal thoracic artery graft.*

With the saphenous technique, as many segments of the vein can be used as necessary, to achieve double or triple bypass grafts (bottom). Sometimes a combination of the two techniques is used, but the thoracic is preferred because the grafts last longer. More than 90 percent of thoracic artery grafts remain unblocked after ten years, compared with 60 percent of vein grafts.

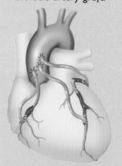

Triple bypass *with saphenous vein grafts.*

The surgical procedure

1 Once the patient is fully anesthetized, the surgeon makes an incision in the chest and uses a saw to cut through the breastbone. The chest is opened with a specialized retractor, which holds the ribs out of the way to allow access to the heart. In the operation shown here, the saphenous vein is being used, so a second surgeon is removing lengths of this vein from the leg.

2 The patient is connected to a heart–lung machine. The aorta is clamped and the heart is injected with a cold potassium solution to stop it from beating. The heart is now still and clear of blood, allowing the surgeons to make the graft.

3 The surgeon sews one end of the saphenous vein segment into a tiny hole cut into the affected coronary artery. The other end is sewn onto the aorta, bypassing the blockage. In the thoracic technique, the surgeon detaches the

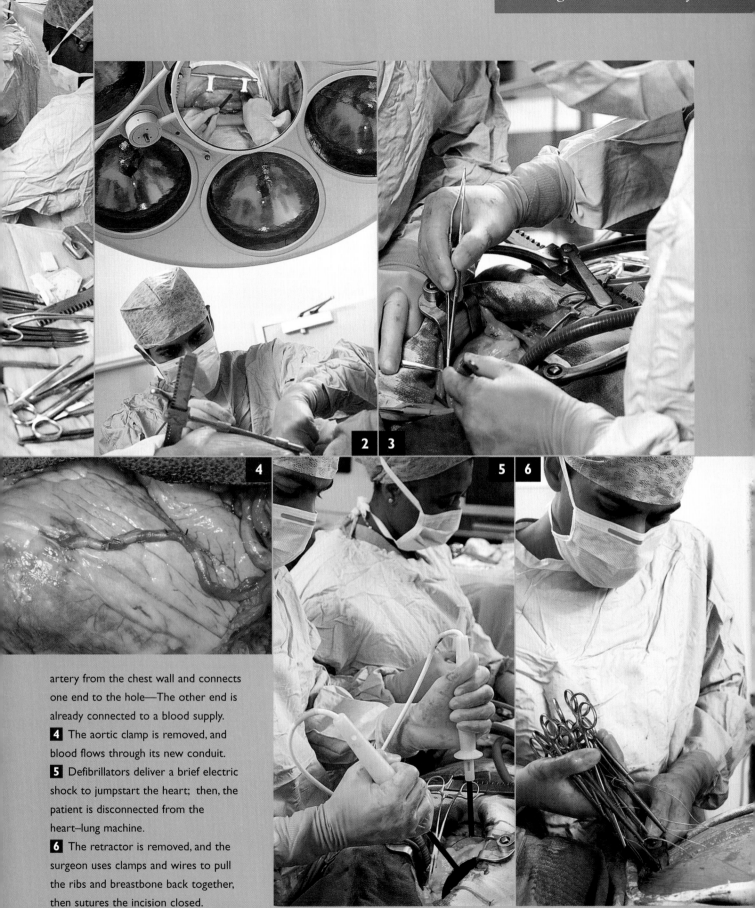

2 3 4 5 6

artery from the chest wall and connects one end to the hole—The other end is already connected to a blood supply.

4 The aortic clamp is removed, and blood flows through its new conduit.

5 Defibrillators deliver a brief electric shock to jumpstart the heart; then, the patient is disconnected from the heart–lung machine.

6 The retractor is removed, and the surgeon uses clamps and wires to pull the ribs and breastbone back together, then sutures the incision closed.

125

A heart-stopping event

Most heart surgery is performed while the heart is temporarily stopped so that surgeons can handle the organ. The heart muscle is stopped with a cold potassium solution, and the heart–lung machine takes over the function of supplying oxygenated blood to the body's tissues. The heart can be stopped and safely operated on for two hours or more. After the operation, the heart is restarted and circulation restored to the patient's own heart and lungs.

The way forward

An increasing number of heart surgeries are performed in a less invasive way through small incisions in the chest or using techniques that avoid the use of the heart–lung machine. Specialized equipment, including thoracoscopic instruments (devices for looking inside the chest) and robotic technology, is used to perform these procedures.

CORONARY ARTERY BYPASS GRAFTING

The coronary arteries commonly become narrowed by a build-up of fat, cholesterol, and other substances as we become older. This process, called atherosclerosis, could slow or stop the flow of blood through the heart's blood vessels. If the flow is reduced, it may cause angina, a very unpleasant crushing or choking sensation in the chest, and if the obstruction completely blocks a vessel, it leads to a heart attack.

Typically, this atherosclerotic narrowing occurs within the first fraction of inch of the major branches feeding the heart. Thus, it is possible to reroute blood into the artery using a bypass graft. Surgeons take a vein from another part of the body, such as the leg or the

AT THE LEADING EDGE

Surgery without stopping the heart

Normally the heart has to be stopped before a surgeon can work on it. In a new technique, however, a special clamp is laid over the blocked artery, holding that region of the heart still enough to operate on, while the rest continues beating. The heart doesn't have to be stopped and use of a heart–lung machine is avoided, reducing the likelihood of complications.

chest, and attach one end to the diseased blood vessel just beyond the blockage and the other end to an artery. The risks attached to this type of surgery are extremely low, although narrowing of the bypass graft occurs in about 1 in every 20 patients.

HEART VALVE SURGERY

The valves between the chambers of the heart are exposed to constant wear and tear, and can also be damaged by infection. As a result, over the course of a lifetime, heart valves can start to leak (a condition known as regurgitation), become narrowed (stenosis), or obstruct normal blood flow. In these cases, doctors may decide to repair or replace the offending valves surgically. The mitral valve (between the two chambers of the left side of the heart), and the aortic valve (which is situated at the outlet of the left ventricle), are those most commonly affected in adults. In order to reach the damaged valve, the surgeon approaches it via one of the atria or major vessels leading to the heart. Whether the valve requires replacement or can be repaired depends on how badly it is damaged. Repair is usually reserved for mitral valves that leak or are narrowed but are not seriously damaged.

Occluded heart

Coronary arteries snake over the surface of the heart in this angiogram, supplying vital oxygen to the hard-working muscle. At the top, however, an occlusion, or total blockage, cutting off the blood supply to one of the arteries, is clearly visible.

Replacement valves

When the valve is to be replaced, the doctor needs to decide what type of replacement valve to use. There is no ideal substitute for the real thing, and selection depends on a variety of factors, including the age of the patient and his or her risk of blood clotting. There are two main types of replacement valves:

- **Mechanical valves** These consist of various combinations of titanium steel, silastic, and now, most commonly, a dense carbon material known as pyrolitic graphite. These are highly durable, but because they are made of artificial materials, there is a greater risk of blood clots developing on their surface. To help prevent this, patients need to take anticoagulant drugs for the rest of their lives. Another side effect of using artificial materials is that they make a clicking sound.

- **Tissue valves** Also called biological valves, these are made from animal tissue. Anticoagulant drugs are needed only for the first few weeks after surgery. Tissue valves do not click, but they are not very durable, and, especially in young adults and children, they tend to wear out after 10 years.

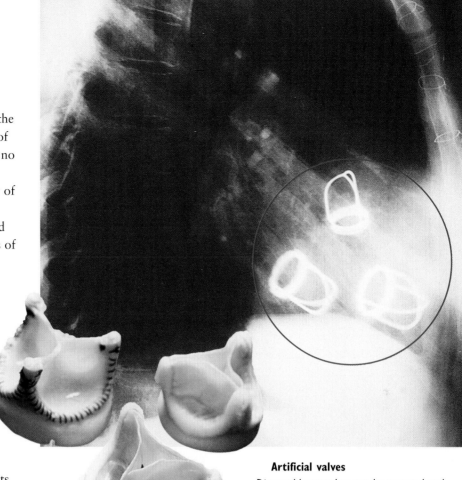

Artificial valves

Diseased heart valves can be removed and replaced with artificial ones. The valves shown on the left are made from pig tissue. The X-ray shows mechanical versions of the aortic, mitral, and tricuspid valves, in place in a man's heart.

What kind of heart valve?

TALKING POINT

The debate about using animal tissue to replace diseased human parts continues. Many people would prefer to receive an artificial valve—either out of principle, or because they dislike the idea of animal tissue inside the human body. Advances in genetic engineering could mean that valves made from pig tissue will soon be superior to artificial ones, but this does raise concerns that new viruses will be able to cross the species barrier.

REPAIR OF CONGENITAL DEFECTS

About 1 in 100 babies is born with a heart defect, most of which can be surgically repaired at some stage during early childhood. The most common of these defects is a "hole in the heart"—a defect in the wall between the two upper or the two lower heart chambers. Some very small holes close spontaneously in the first year of life. Larger holes, however, need to be repaired; otherwise, blood mixes in the chambers and can cause serious problems.

Closing "hole in the heart" defects usually involves open heart surgery and the use of a heart–lung machine. In order to reach the hole, the surgeon needs to cut open the heart, and then sew together or patch the defect (using a square of artificial material or a graft from the membrane surrounding the heart). One technique developed recently avoids the need for invasive surgery: A device is threaded up to the heart through blood vessels and is implanted in the defect. Using this technique, some children are actually able to return home within one to two days of surgery.

TRANSPLANTATION

Heart and heart–lung transplantation have improved considerably in recent years but are carried out only when a disease is irreversible and life-threatening and has not responded to any other treatment. In the United States, a patient's doctor completes a United Network for Organ Sharing (Unet) form, and the patient, given a beeper, joins the 67,000 people on the organ waiting list. Each is classified by medical need. During the transplantations, surgeons remove the diseased organs and replace them with healthy ones taken from a person who has recently died. Currently, very few heart and heart–lung transplants are carried out, mainly due to a lack of donors.

For those lucky enough to receive a transplant, the long-term outlook is now good. Between 85 and 90 percent of transplant patients live for at least a year after the transplant; 75 percent are alive after 5 years, and between 50 and 60 percent are still alive after 10 years.

Heart transplant patients can be up and about remarkably quickly— sometimes within four days of their operation.

THE ROAD TO RECOVERY

Almost certainly, a person who has had heart or major vascular surgery, particularly if a heart–lung bypass machine was used, will spend a short period of time (usually about 24 hours) in an intensive care unit (ICU) before returning to the cardiac ward.

The mass of equipment in the ICU can appear intimidating to patients and their families, but most of it is for routine purposes. Tubes connected to the wrist allow blood monitoring, and a catheter removes urine from the bladder and checks its content. At first there may be a tube down the patient's throat, attached to a ventilator, to help with breathing. Later, oxygen and water vapor may be supplied via a mask.

The patient is started on a rehabilitation programme as soon as possible. During this time, it is quite common for anxiety or depression to set in for a few days, as a natural consequence of the stressful events, but it's surprising how quickly a person regains confidence, especially with support from family and friends.

A full recovery from major surgery usually takes about three months. On average, a patient can leave the hospital about five days after heart surgery, but it usually takes another three weeks to feel stronger and regain normal body habits. Many people can return to employment within six weeks. Heavy work, however, should be avoided for the first three months, and driving a car is not recommended for at least four weeks.

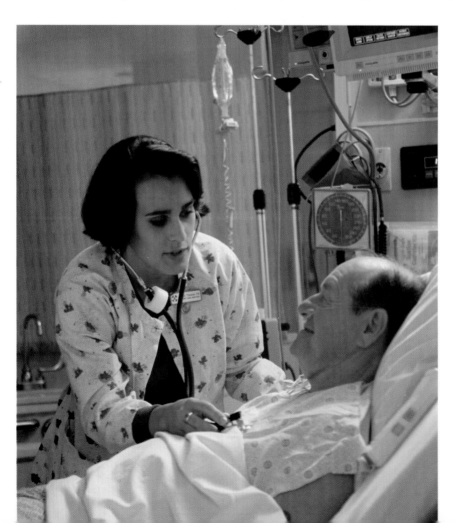

The intensive care unit
Operated by highly experienced and qualified staff, the ICU is also known as the cardiac recovery unit, cardiothoracic surgical unit, or intensive therapy unit, depending on the hospital. Here postoperative patients are carefully monitored to ensure rapid recovery.

Surgical repair of blood vessels

The range of operations within the vascular surgeon's repertoire is astonishing, extending from routine varicose vein removal to life-saving surgery to repair a ruptured aortic aneurysm— a defect in the body's main artery.

REPAIR OF AN AORTIC ANEURYSM

The aorta is the main arterial highway, running from the left side of the heart down the length of the abdomen. It is responsible for carrying oxygenated blood to the entire body and is large, strong, and elastic. Sometimes, however, a weakness develops in the walls of the artery, known as an aneurysm, and the vessel "balloons out," This bulging most often occurs within the abdominal section of the aorta. If an aneurysm bursts, it could have potentially fatal consequences, so any defect measuring more than 2½ inches in diameter is repaired surgically.

> **Someone with an aortic aneurysm may suffer acute chest pain and think they are having a heart attack.**

The operation

An aortic aneurysm repair is a major surgical procedure and as such is only carried out if absolutely necessary. Even so, the operation is fairly straightforward.

First, the surgeon makes a 6-inch incision in the abdomen. Once the aneurysm is located, a bypass is put in place using an artificial blood vessel, known as a prosthetic graft. This tubular graft is slipped inside the

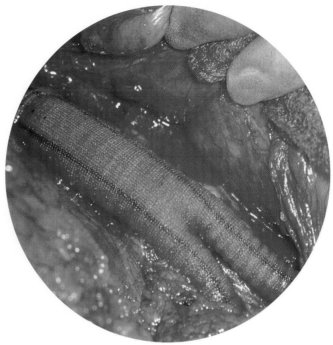

Aortic graft in place
If an aneurysm occurs where the aorta branches into the femoral arteries, surgeons repair the damage with a "trouser graft," so-called because the prosthetic blood vessel splits into two branches.

aorta at the site of weakness and stitched top and bottom to hold it securely in place. With time, the normal lining cells of the aorta grow on the inner surface of the graft, giving a long-lasting conduit for blood to flow through.

After surgery

Once the operation is completed, it's usual to have a day's stay in the intensive care unit. On average, a patient is discharged home after 7 to 10 days in hospital.

VARICOSE VEIN REMOVAL

If the valves within veins that help blood flow back toward the heart are weak or fail, the changed blood flow pattern can cause distortion in these vessels, resulting in varicose veins. Unsightly varicose veins can be distressing and painful. Left untreated, they can lead to complications such as deep vein thrombosis. The problem can be rectified with surgery, but there are other

AT THE LEADING EDGE

Repairing vessels from within

Techniques to carry out aortic aneurysm repair without the need for open surgery—endovascular repairs—are currently undergoing trials, and initial results are extremely promising. The graft is inserted into an artery in the groin, passed up to the aorta, and opened out inside the aneurysm. Tiny attaching mechanisms clip onto the artery wall above and below the aneurysm to secure the graft in place. No incisions are made, so a hospital stay can be as short as two days.

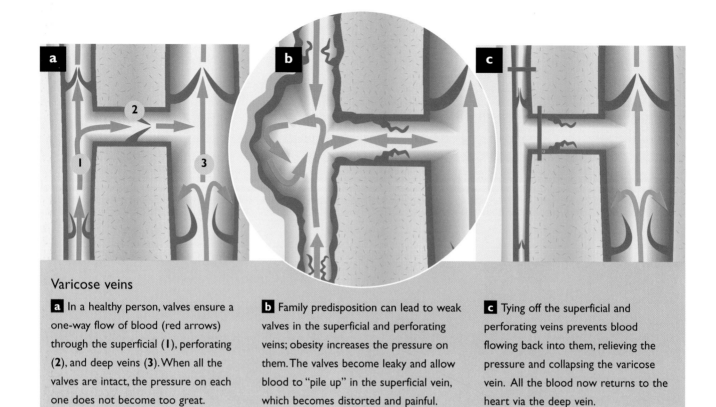

Varicose veins

a In a healthy person, valves ensure a one-way flow of blood (red arrows) through the superficial (**1**), perforating (**2**), and deep veins (**3**). When all the valves are intact, the pressure on each one does not become too great.

b Family predisposition can lead to weak valves in the superficial and perforating veins; obesity increases the pressure on them. The valves become leaky and allow blood to "pile up" in the superficial vein, which becomes distorted and painful.

c Tying off the superficial and perforating veins prevents blood flowing back into them, relieving the pressure and collapsing the varicose vein. All the blood now returns to the heart via the deep vein.

treatment methods, such as injection of an irritant fluid to make the inside walls of the veins stick together. Doctors will recommend a procedure based on the severity of the varicose veins. Surgical removal of the offending veins can be over and done with in less than a day, and is generally extremely effective.

The operation

Beforehand, the surgeon draws around the affected veins on the patient's leg while standing up. Once in the operating room with the patient under a general anesthetic, small incisions—about 2 inches long—are made in the groin and just behind the knee. The long saphenous vein, which runs down the length of the leg, is withdrawn from the thigh to avoid recurrence of varicose veins. The dilated veins are then removed through tiny stab wounds in the legs. Once the tiny holes are stitched up, the leg is carefully pressure-bandaged.

The whole operation takes less than an hour, and a patient is usually allowed home the next day. Because the incisions are so small, there is very little scarring. Afterwards, patients are advised to wear supportive elastic stockings to encourage healthy blood flow through the veins in the legs.

CAROTID ENDARTERECTOMY

If the artery supplying blood to the brain becomes clogged up because of atherosclerosis, there is high risk of a stroke occurring. Surgical removal of the blockage can be carried out under either general or local anesthetic and is a delicate and skilled procedure.

The operation

An incision is made in the neck, and the blocked artery is clipped and opened out so that the fatty plaque can be cut away. During the operation, a piece of tubing called a shunt is placed inside the artery so that oxygenated blood can flow through it and continue to supply the brain, while the surgeon is working on the plaque.

Recovery from a carotid endarterectomy takes two to three days; complications are rare, although occasionally a stroke can occur during or immediately after surgery. Currently, experts are looking into relieving carotid artery blockage using balloon angioplasty (see page 119), but this technique is not yet routine.

Recovering from a heart attack

After a heart attack, the time spent in the hospital is relatively short. The journey begins when the crisis is over and the person has to consider how to adapt to a new lifestyle. A positive attitude and support from family and friends make the transition easier and more successful.

POSITIVE THINKING

A heart attack can have long-lasting implications. Although many people recover completely, a structured rehabilitation program cuts the risk of needing to be readmitted to the hospital by half and is crucial for a smooth return to normal life. It also helps to instill optimism about the future and boost confidence. Fears about subsequent attacks are inevitable, and a person needs to overcome any anxieties about resuming an active lifestyle. Experts have consistently proved that a person with a positive mental attitude will recover more quickly and return to work earlier than those who are less determined.

THE REHABILITATION PROCESS

The process of recovery begins in the hospital, very soon after a heart attack. In most cases, there are three main areas of rehabilitation: education about heart disease and its prevention, dietary modification, and exercise programs. Many cardiac units—wards that specialize in heart disease—have formalized rehabilitation programs and will, at the very least, distribute information leaflets. It has been consistently shown that a better informed patient is more likely to comply with ongoing treatments or lifestyle changes.

The role of education

Rehabilitation can involve major lifestyle adjustments to reduce the impact of the risk factors that contributed to the heart attack in the first place. In most hospitals, patients receive education about the causes of heart attacks, the drugs that they will need to take in the long term, and the steps they need to take to reduce the chances of a second attack. Stopping smoking is the single most effective measure that a smoker can take to reduce the chances of having another attack. The improvement in survival after cessation of smoking compares very favorably with the benefits obtained from more "high-

Continued smoking after a heart attack doubles the chance of having another attack. Giving up can halve the risk within two years.

tech" therapies such as angioplasty or coronary artery bypass surgery. Individual counseling and support of the patient is probably the most successful approach, and most cardiac rehabilitation programs incorporate a smoking-cessation module.

The week after a heart attack

Most people who have a heart attack stay in the hospital for five to seven days. During this time, cardiac nurses initiate a "schedule" of activities to speed recovery and remobilize the patient, so that a brief hospital stay is possible.

NUMBER OF DAYS AFTERWARD	
1	Sit up and walk a few steps around the bed. Do breathing exercises in bed.
2	Get up aided and take short walks through the room and to the bathroom.
3	Continue as Day 2 but with less help and supervision.
4	Walk with the physical therapist along the corridor and up and down the stairs.
5	As Day 4.
6	Continue walking farther; possibly go home.
7	Go home.

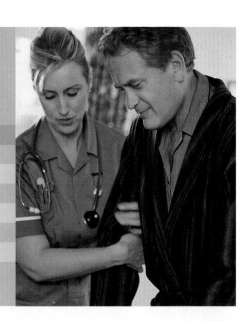

Eating for life

There is plenty of evidence to show that people who eat a diet low in saturated fats and cholesterol have less of a risk of developing heart disease. Therefore, it is not surprising that patients who have already had a heart attack also benefit from modification of their diet to reduce saturated fat intake. Protection for patients with heart disease is complex, however; it is not guaranteed simply because of a reduction in the level of blood fats. Current guidelines recommend that patients who have had a heart attack should increase their consumption of fresh fruit and vegetables to at least five portions per day.

Getting going again

A gradual increase in physical activity is an important part of the rehabilitation program. Individual exercise schedules are usually supervised by cardiac nurses and physical therapists until the patient has reached a particular level of physical activity safely. Exercise has many benefits for someone who has had a heart attack:

- Improvements in lung function and blood pressure
- An increase in "good" (HDL) cholesterol and a decrease in "bad" (LDL) cholesterol
- A reduction in the "stickiness" of the blood platelets involved in clotting and increases in the levels of the body's natural clot-dissolving substances

Is it all right to have sex after a heart attack?

Sexual activity after a heart attack should be viewed in the same light as any physical exercise and does not put any "extra" strain on the heart. The same rules should be followed as for any exercise: If sexual intercourse brings on chest pain or severe breathlessness, stop and rest for a few minutes. With time, most people will be able to resume a normal sex life, but, as with exercise, it is important to start slowly.

ASK THE EXPERT

- The formation of new blood vessels that grow into the damaged area of heart muscle and improve the blood supply (and consequently deliver more oxygen)

Patients recovering from a heart attack are sometimes tempted to engage in overvigorous physical activity too soon. This is why a doctor-supervised program is preferable, because it moderates overenthusiasm on the part of the patient. Regular exercise can take many forms and people usually find the activity that suits them best. Walking or swimming are both excellent ways to improve aerobic fitness and are normally encouraged.

Physical activity can sometimes bring on an episode of chest pain or breathlessness. If this happens, stop exercising until the pain has abated; if the pain does not resolve after 5 to 10 minutes, take some of the nitrate spray prescribed or pop a tablet under your tongue. If the spray is ineffective, seek urgent medical advice.

WHAT DOES THE FUTURE HOLD?

Having a heart attack is not the end of the world; the majority of people make a full recovery and resume normal living, albeit with some limitations. High-tech medicines and therapies can achieve only so much—Most people will need to make major lifestyle changes after a heart attack to aid in full recovery and to reduce the chances of developing any further cardiac problems.

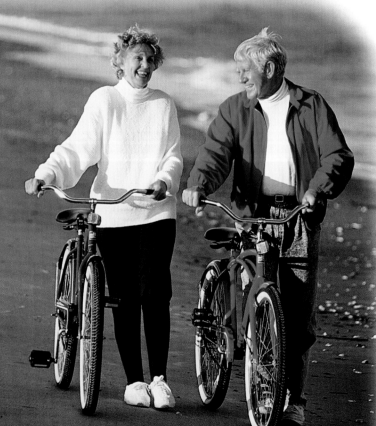

The road to recovery
A heart attack can be a warning—a stimulus to adopt a new approach to exercise, diet, and lifestyle, one that improves all-round quality of life, while protecting cardiovascular health.

A TO Z

OF DISEASES AND DISORDERS

This section gives information on the main illnesses and medical conditions that affect the heart and circulatory system. Entries are arranged alphabetically, and each entry is structured in a similar way:

What are the causes?

What are the symptoms?

How is it diagnosed?

What are the treatment options?

What is the outlook?

How can it be prevented or minimized?

ANGINA
See Coronary artery disease, p. 137.

AORTIC ANEURYSM
A weakness in the wall of the main artery of the body that causes it to expand like a balloon under pressure.

The aorta is the largest and most important artery of the body. It stretches from the heart to the lower abdomen and carries oxygenated blood under high pressure. Normally, the strong elastic walls of the aorta cope with this pressure, but in some people an area becomes weakened. The pressure generated by the pumping heart causes the aorta to progressively expand the area where the vessel wall is weak; eventually the aneurysm may become so large and damaged that it may leak or even burst. Any part of the artery may be affected, but the most common site is where the aorta passes through the abdomen.

What are the causes?
Most aortic aneurysms are due to atherosclerosis, the formation of fatty plaques on the inside of the artery walls. Among the factors that contribute to atherosclerosis are smoking, a high-fat diet, and high blood pressure. Experts believe that there may be a genetic element to the condition because there is a tendency for abdominal aortic aneurysms to run in families. In a small number of cases, aneurysms may be caused by trauma, inflammation, infection, or congenital abnormalities of the arterial wall.

What are the symptoms?
In many cases, an aortic aneurysm does not cause any symptoms. If large, an abdominal aneurysm can cause pain or discomfort in the lower back or stomach. Aneurysms higher up the aorta in the chest (thoracic aneurysms) are also usually asymptomatic, although some people experience chest pain. Sometimes, the aneurysm becomes so large that it starts to leak blood or bursts, causing a breach in the arterial wall. In these cases, sudden severe stomach and back pain is common and the loss of blood results in shock. A ruptured aneurysm can be fatal if the breach in the aorta is large.

How is it diagnosed?
Because of the lack of symptoms, aortic aneurysms are often discovered only during a visit to a doctor for another reason. During a medical examination, the doctor may notice a pulsating swelling in the abdomen, which could indicate an abdominal aortic aneurysm. Doctors use Doppler ultrasound scanning (p. 109) or computed tomography (CT) scanning to confirm the presence of an aneurysm and to assess its size. Thoracic aortic aneurysms can be diagnosed from a chest X-ray (p. 105), although echocardiography (p. 106) or CT scanning are usually carried out to assess the size of the problem.

What are the treatment options?
Generally, aortic aneurysms are repaired by surgery to replace or bypass the damaged section of artery with a synthetic graft (p. 129). If an aneurysm is leaking or has ruptured, surgery is usually an emergency. In other situations, the operation is performed only if the aneurysm becomes large, making a rupture more likely to occur.

How can it be prevented or minimized?
Living a healthy lifestyle to reduce the risk of developing atherosclerosis is one of the best ways to prevent both the development and the progression of an aortic aneurysm. In people with a strong family history of aneurysms or conditions known to be associated with their development, screening with ultrasound or CT may be carried out to allow early detection of potential sites of aneurysm.

ATHEROSCLEROSIS
A build-up of fatty deposits on the interior of artery walls; it primarily affects the body's major arteries, where there is high pressure and turbulent blood flow.

The word atherosclerosis derives from Greek—*athere* meaning porridge and *skleros* meaning hardening. It is the clogging of arteries by deposits of plaque, which is made of atheroma—a mixture of cholesterol, decaying muscle cells, fibrous tissue, clumps of blood platelets, and sometimes calcium. Plaque formation narrows the arteries so blood can't get through to supply oxygen and nutrients. Ultimately, the affected area of the body—commonly the heart, legs, or head—simply starves. Atherosclerosis of the coronary arteries leads to coronary artery disease.

Atherosclerosis is responsible for more deaths in the United States and most other Western countries than any other condition.

What are the causes?
Fatty substances including cholesterol, also known as lipids, are transported in the blood, bound together with proteins to form particles called lipoproteins. If there is too

much cholesterol in a person's bloodstream, the cholesterol begins to build up in the form of low-density lipoproteins (LDLs). LDLs are sticky and sometimes adhere to the insides of blood vessel walls, particularly in medium-sized and large arteries. Because they contribute to plaque formation, LDLs are often referred to as "bad" cholesterol. High-density lipoproteins—HDLs—are known as "good" cholesterol.

The plaque build-up results from a combination of excess lipids and damage to blood vessel walls (by high blood pressure or turbulent flow). White blood cells responding to artery damage stick to the vessel lining and release chemicals to attract other cells to "heal" the injured blood vessel. So, the previously smooth artery lining starts to develop streaks of sticky plaques, which attract more plaque and cause turbulence—and a vicious circle begins.

Factors that increase a person's risk of developing atherosclerosis include the following:

- Smoking
- A family history of atherosclerosis
- Diabetes mellitus or high blood pressure
- Being overweight
- A high blood cholesterol level
- An inactive lifestyle

Personality type and how well a person copes with stress can also have a bearing on the development of atherosclerosis; having an aggressive personality and not being able to manage stress effectively is thought to increase the risk of this disease.

What are the symptoms?

Unfortunately, atherosclerosis produces no symptoms until the damage to the arteries is severe enough to restrict blood flow. Symptoms caused by progressive atherosclerotic narrowing of an artery are more likely to occur during exercise than at rest, at least initially. Early symptoms may occur only after great exertion, but as the narrowing worsens, less and less activity is required to produce the same response. The specific symptoms depend on the artery or arteries obstructed:

- Restriction of blood flow to the heart muscle can cause chest pain (angina) or even a heart attack
- If arteries in the legs are affected, then symptoms include numbness, fatigue, and pain in the leg—known as intermittent claudication.
- Narrowing of the arteries supplying blood to the brain may cause transient ischemic attacks (symptoms and signs of a stroke lasting fewer than 24 hours) and episodes of dizziness.

Aspirin—the inexpensive wonderdrug?

TALKING POINT

Numerous research studies have confirmed the benefits of aspirin in preventing heart attacks and strokes in people with atherosclerosis. So should a daily dose of the drug be a routine part of life for anyone over 50? In fact, experts continue to disagree about whether the drug is actually effective in the prevention of heart disease in people with no symptoms. Doctors are increasingly wary about prescribing drugs as a preventative measure, primarily because the drugs themselves may have side effects. In the case of aspirin, although the drug effectively thins the blood, helping to prevent hazardous clots from forming, it can also increase the risk of spontaneous bleeding. Generally, however, aspirin has few side effects, although it is not recommended for people with stomach problems such as gastric ulcers.

How is it diagnosed?

A medical history and examination (p. 98) will reveal much about the health of the circulation, but special investigations may be necessary. Possible tests include measurement of blood lipids (p. 102) and investigation of arterial blood flow by angiography (p. 109) or, for the legs or peripheral circulation, Doppler ultrasound scanning (p. 109).

What are the treatment options?

There is encouraging data to suggest that a major decrease in blood cholesterol level, accomplished through lipid-lowering drugs, diet, and other lifestyle changes, can slow, and in a few cases reverse, plaque build-up.

- To minimize secondary clotting (the thinking behind "an aspirin a day"), doctors may prescribe anticoagulant drugs (p. 115).
- Symptoms are relieved in many people by vasodilators (p. 116), drugs that widen narrowed blood vessels.
- Surgical treatment (p. 122) may be recommended for people who are unresponsive to medication or who have a high risk of suffering serious complications. Balloon angioplasty (p. 119) may be used to open up narrowed vessels. Atheroma can be removed by endarterectomy (p. 130) and segments of diseased peripheral vessels can be replaced by woven plastic tube grafts (p. 129).

How can it be prevented or minimized?

To prevent any recurrence of a major episode, patients are recommended to give up smoking, get regular exercise, and eat a low-cholesterol, low-fat diet.

BRADYCARDIA
An abnormally slow heartbeat.

A healthy heartbeat varies widely during the day, depending upon activity and level of fitness. Athletes at peak physical condition can have a heart rate as low as 40—a rate that is an indication of fitness in a healthy person and is of no concern. Doctors diagnose bradycardia when, because of disease or old age, the heart slows down to a rate lower than is normal for a particular individual.

What are the causes?

There is a range of causes for bradycardia. It is sometimes a reaction to a sudden emotional shock or severe pain and often occurs in association with fainting. In older people, the natural pacemaker of the heart, which generates the electrical impulses that cause the heart to beat, may not work properly, leading to periods when the heart slows or even stops for a few seconds for no apparent reason. Both old age and coronary artery disease can prevent the electrical signals from reaching the pumping chambers of the heart—the ventricles. When this happens, the ventricles continue to beat, but at a much slower rate, a condition known as complete heart block. Sometimes the drugs used to treat heart conditions can themselves interfere with the function of the heart's electrical system and slow the rate.

What are the symptoms?

Bradycardia may come on intermittently so that the symptoms occur only every now and then, or it can be continuous and unrelenting. Commonly experienced symptoms include the following:

• A sensation of lightheadedness, as if one is about to faint
• An awareness of a slow, heavy heartbeat
• Loss of consciousness, which is brief and usually without warning
• Shortness of breath

If a very slow heartbeat continues for a period of time, a person can become very unwell. Eventually shock will develop, in which the body's organs are not receiving enough blood, requiring life-saving treatment.

How is it diagnosed?

The diagnosis hinges upon capturing the abnormal heart rate during an examination and on an electrocardiogram (ECG)—a tracing of the electrical activity of the heart (p. 103). This is easy if the bradycardia is persistent, but it can be problematic if the heart rate slows intermittently. An ECG may need to be monitored over a period of 24 hours or more to detect the abnormality.

What are the treatment options?

The treatment for bradycardia depends on the cause of the problem and its severity. If a person's heartbeat is so slow that it is causing symptoms of shock, the doctor will immediately administer a drug intravenously (atropine and/or isoadrenaline) to speed up the heart rate. If this fails, a temporary pacemaker may be required to restore a normal rate. This treatment involves placing wires directly into the heart muscle and passing small electrical impulses down them so that the ventricles contract. If the bradycardia persists, a permanent pacemaker (p. 121) can be inserted under the skin. Intermittent bradycardias associated with age or disease may require a permanent pacemaker if severe or if they cause troublesome symptoms. When a bradycardia is caused by a drug, switching to a different type of drug usually restores a normal rhythm.

CARDIOMYOPATHY
Damage to the heart muscle leading to enlargement of the heart or thickening of the heart muscle.

The heart is fundamentally a single powerful muscle that sends blood coursing through the body with every contraction. If the muscle tissue is directly damaged, the heart can become enlarged and floppy so that its ability to act as a pump is impaired—a condition known as cardiomyopathy. There are two main types: dilated and hypertrophic. Dilated cardiomyopathy, where the heart muscle stretches and weakens, is the most common. Hypertrophic cardiomyopathy is much more rare and particularly affects the left ventricle, the walls of which become abnormally thickened.

What are the causes?

The causes of cardiomyopathy are not well understood. Although a range of problems are linked with the disorder, it is not always clear exactly how they lead to the damaging changes to heart tissue. Dilated cardiomyopathy is linked to alcohol abuse, or it may result from an autoimmune condition, where the body's immune system attacks its own tissues. Some viral infections can also cause rapid severe damage to heart muscle, often in young adults or children, and although in many instances the damage is reversible, this is not always the case.

There are many other causes including diseases of the heart valves, infections, and hereditary disorders—In most cases hypertrophic cardiomyopathy is an inherited problem. High blood pressure is also linked to heart muscle disease. Over months or years, heart muscle becomes thickened and eventually becomes less able to perform its function. In some cases of cardiomyopathy, doctors are unable to discover a specific cause.

What are the symptoms?

As cardiomyopathy progresses, the heart becomes unable to function properly, and symptoms of heart failure begin to develop. Initially, a person with cardiomyopathy may have no symptoms at all, particularly if the damage to the heart muscle is minimal. When the damage is more severe, the symptoms include the following:

Night-time can bring on symptoms for many people who are unable to lie flat without feeling short of breath and have to increase the number of pillows to give a more upright position for sleeping.

• Breathlessness on exertion
• Swelling of the lower legs
• Fatigue
• Loss of appetite

People with long-standing cardiomyopathy may noticeably begin to lose weight.

How is it diagnosed?

A physical examination (p. 98) may give the doctor a strong indication of the diagnosis, although when the heart muscle disease is mild, very little evidence can be found, especially in people who lead a fairly sedentary lifestyle. Although a tracing of the electrical activity of the heart—an electrocardiogram (p. 103)—and chest X-ray (p. 105) may support the diagnosis, the most efficient investigation for suspected heart muscle damage is the echocardiogram (p. 106). Not only will this investigation confirm the diagnosis, in many cases it can provide clues as to the initial cause of the cardiomyopathy.

Further investigations are directed toward finding any evidence of an underlying disorder, and may involve exercise treadmill testing (p. 104), cardiac catheterization (p. 110), and biopsy of the heart muscle, in addition to a variety of blood tests (p. 102).

What are the treatment options?

Many of the causes of cardiomyopathy are treatable, and, if diagnosed early, treatment can slow the progression of heart muscle damage. If the condition is caused by hypertension, and the muscle has become thickened but has not started to fail, effective treatment of blood pressure can sometimes reverse the damage. In those with alcohol-related damage, there may be a striking recovery with time if drinking is stopped. Surgical repair or replacement of diseased valves will prevent further damage but often does little to reverse existing changes.

Symptoms of heart failure caused by cardiomyopathy may be teated with drugs such as diuretics and ACE inhibitors (p.114), and there is good evidence that in such cases drug therapy helps to prevent any further decline in heart muscle function. If the damage to the heart muscle is very severe, especially in younger people, heart transplantation (p. 128) may be considered.

What is the outlook?

The outlook for people with cardiomyopathy depends very much on the cause of the problem. In general, though, if muscle damage is severe, the outlook is poor, especially if the symptoms of heart failure have developed.

CORONARY ARTERY DISEASE

Damage to or malfunction of the heart caused by narrowing or blockage of the coronary arteries, the vessels that supply blood to the heart muscle.

The exact causes of coronary disease remain obscure, but it is almost exclusively a disease of the Western world. A number of risk factors have been identified that make it more likely that a person will develop coronary disease: increasing age, male gender, cigarette smoking, high cholesterol, high blood pressure, diabetes, and a family history of premature heart disease. However, many people who suffer heart attack do not have any of these risk factors. Experts are researching possible new causes, such as the common bacterium *Chlamydia* or increased levels of chemicals, such as homocysteine, in the blood.

What are the symptoms?

In most people, the primary symptom of coronary artery disease is chest pain—angina. Angina develops most commonly during exercise when the blood flow through the narrowed arteries is unable to satisfy the heart muscle's increased demand for oxygen. The pain is often described as a heavy pressure that starts in the center of the chest but that can radiate down the left arm or up to the lower jaw. If the pain continues at rest and is particularly severe, it may indicate that a person is having a heart attack, or myocardial infarction. In this case, an artery has become completely blocked, so the area of heart muscle supplied by that artery dies.

Some people, particularly the elderly and those with diabetes, may not experience chest pain, making the diagnosis of angina or a heart attack difficult. These people often develop heart failure as a result of progressive damage to the heart muscle, which causes breathlessness and ankle swelling.

HELP YOUR DOCTOR TO HELP YOU

Describing chest pain

If you suffer an episode of chest pain, seek medical attention. The doctor will ask a series of questions to try to ascertain if the pain is originating from the heart, and it will help to consider the answers to these questions.

- *When did the pain begin and what were you doing at the time? For example, were you exercising or at rest?*

- *How did the pain come on—Was it gradual or sudden?*

- *How would you describe the pain? Consider its location (central chest, back, arms, jaw); the nature of the pain (heavy, dull, ache); and its severity ("worst pain ever experienced," constant, intermittent).*

- *Is there anything that relieves the pain or makes it worse, such as changing posture or taking an indigestion tablet?*

- *Have you ever had pain of a similar nature before?*

- *Can you identify what triggered the pain?*

- *What other symptoms are you experiencing? Possibilities include breathlessness, sweating, nausea, vomiting, palpitations, total exhaustion, and lightheadedness.*

How is it diagnosed?

Most episodes of chest pain are due to other, less serious causes, such as indigestion or muscle aches, but some are due to heart disease. Doctors, therefore, need to know whether a patient might have coronary artery disease before carrying out invasive tests that could place him or her at risk. They have devised strategies to help make this decision, based on a thorough medical history and physical examination. In addition, an exercise ECG (p. 104), radionuclide perfusion imaging (p. 108), or stress echocardiography (p. 107) may be carried out to provide extra clues as to the cause of the chest pain. The results of these tests help the doctor to decide whether a patient should go on to have coronary angiography (p. 109).

What are the treatment options?

People with coronary artery disease are treated with an array of drugs and procedures based on evidence gathered from some of the largest scientific studies ever carried out. For each individual, the most suitable treatment depends on the severity of the symptoms, which can range from slight breathlessness to a serious heart attack.

Regular exercise significantly reduces the likelihood of developing CAD.

- **Drug therapy** It is now recommended that everyone with coronary artery disease takes a small dose of aspirin each day to impair blood clotting slightly, which reduces the risk of a heart attack. If the cholesterol level in the blood is even slightly raised, doctors may prescribe a drug called a statin (p. 115). Some people with heart disease may benefit from ACE inhibitor drugs, which are usually used to treat people with high blood pressure or heart failure. Drugs for angina (p. 116) include a spray of nitroglycerin, or tiny tablets that can be placed under the tongue, to relieve or prevent individual episodes by dilating the arteries that supply the heart muscle. If the symptoms are frequent, beta-blockers, often in combination with nitrates or calcium antagonists, may be prescribed as a preventative measure.

- **Angioplasty** People who continue to experience angina despite medication, or who are thought to have a high risk of a future heart attack, may undergo balloon angioplasty (p. 119) to widen the affected blood vessels.

- **Surgery** If all three of the main coronary arteries are affected, or if there is a narrowing in the main stem of the left coronary artery, coronary artery bypass graft surgery (p. 124) may be necessary to provide an alternative route for the blood supply.

What is the outlook?

The main concern for people with coronary artery disease is the risk of a future or second heart attack—the outcome of which is fatal in more than half of all cases. The more severe the disease, the greater the risk of a heart attack.

How can it be prevented or minimized?

Living a healthy lifestyle, exercising regularly, and avoiding high-fat foods and smoking can, to some extent, minimize the risk of heart disease. If there is a strong family history of the condition, doctors may begin regular screening. Once heart disease is diagnosed, doctors will give advice on how to lose weight, if necessary, and on dietary requirements and strategies to stop smoking.

DEEP VEIN THROMBOSIS

Formation of a blood clot (thrombosis) that blocks a vein deep within the muscles of the legs or pelvis, causing swelling and pain.

In this common condition, a vein lying deep within the muscles of one leg (occasionally both) or pelvis becomes blocked by a blood clot, restricting the blood flow. Although, with time, the body usually dissolves the clot, there is a danger that a tiny fragment could break away from the main clot and travel in the bloodstream to the lungs. If large enough, it may block an artery—a life-threatening condition known as a pulmonary embolism.

What are the causes?

In both the leg and the pelvis there are three factors that contribute to the development of deep vein thrombosis. Each may cause a thrombosis on its own, but quite frequently they are all involved to some extent.

- **Damage to the lining of the vein** This may occur following trauma or infection, which acts as an intense stimulus for blood to clot in the affected area.
- **Increased tendency to clot easily** In association with some diseases, blood may clot too easily, leading to a greater tendency for thrombosis. Taking estrogen-containing contraceptives increases the likelihood of this happening.
- **Reduction in venous blood flow** One major cause is inactivity, as may occur during illness, travel, or following an operation. This situation is exacerbated by dehydration, which is why people should drink plenty of nonalcoholic fluids on long trips. Varicose veins may also lead to reduction in venous flow.

EXPERIENCING DEEP VEIN THROMBOSIS

I'm a nurse by profession and had heard about people developing clots on long-distance airline flights, but I never thought it would happen to me, especially because I was always careful.

I was flying to Australia to visit my family, and about halfway through the journey I started to get an achey feeling just below the knee. By the time we were nearing the end of the flight, it felt hot to the touch, and my leg looked red and swollen. I realized that I might have a clot and arranged to see a doctor immediately on landing.

The doctor told me that I had actually developed a deep vein thrombosis, even though I had been careful to drink plenty of water and move about during the long flight. He suggested that being on the contraceptive pill may have contributed. I was quickly admitted to the hospital and given anticoagulant drugs.

What are the symptoms?

A deep vein thrombosis can be present without any symptoms at all. More frequently, though, a variable combination of pain, tenderness, swelling, and purple-red skin discoloration occurs, affecting the calf or thigh of one or both legs, depending upon the level of the blockage. When the blockage is below the knee, pain may be felt only when the person is upright. The skin is often warm to the touch, and the veins on the surface of the leg may be more prominent as blood finds alternative routes along the limb.

How is it diagnosed?

Although a doctor may suspect a deep vein thrombosis on examining the leg, it is necessary to confirm its presence and locate the level and extent of the clot. The simplest way to do this is with a Doppler ultrasound scan (p. 109) of the veins in the legs and pelvis, which can detect the movement of blood. If doctors are still uncertain about the diagnosis, a venogram is performed (p. 109). In this procedure radiopaque dye is injected into the veins of the leg, and X-ray images are taken to locate the clot.

Once the diagnosis is confirmed, blood tests to check clotting ability and further scans to investigate any underlying condition are often required.

What are the treatment options?

To avoid the possibility of a pulmonary embolism, a suspected deep vein thrombosis is treated rapidly with injections of a drug called heparin, which reduces blood clotting. Once the diagnosis is confirmed, another anticoagulant—coumadin—is prescribed in tablet form; these take a few days to reach a therapeutic level in the bloodstream, so the heparin injections are continued until this happens. Drug treatment usually continues for about six months. Since reducing the ability of the blood to clot can lead to abnormal bleeding, monitoring with blood tests at an anticoagulation clinic is required. Even so, people taking warfarin should be aware that they will bleed more easily and should carry a card to inform others of their treatment in the case of an emergency.

Lifelong treatment with coumadin may be necessary if a deep vein thrombosis recurs.

What is the outlook?

Anticoagulation reduces the risk of pulmonary embolism to a minimum, although it may still occur, more usually with very large blood clots. The second major risk results from the restricted blood flow in the leg, which, in a minority of people, continues in the long term after the initial illness. Chronic symptoms of pain, skin discoloration, and swelling may eventually be followed by the formation of leg ulcers. Wearing elastic stockings early on encourages the flow of venous blood from the legs back to the heart and helps to reduce the chance of this complication.

EMBOLISM
Blockage of arteries by abnormally large objects, such as fragments of a blood clot, that form within the circulation and travel in the bloodstream.

Normally, blood flows smoothly through the circulatory system. Sometimes, however, a substance that is not normally present in the circulation—such as a clot, air, or fat—forms within the blood. These substances are known as emboli and, if large enough, they can block arteries and cut off the blood supply to a particular part of the body—a condition known as embolism. If an embolus originates in the veins, it travels back to the right side of the heart and from there into the lungs, where blockage and pulmonary embolism may occur. If the embolus originates in the arteries, it may travel to any part of the body; common sites include the brain, kidney, spleen, intestine, and limbs.

What are the causes?

Emboli come in various types and most of them arise because of an existing medical condition.

- **Blood clot** This is the most common type of embolus. It usually breaks off from an existing clot (thrombus) on the wall of an artery, generally a result of atherosclerosis. A clot embolus may originate in the heart: Thrombi often form on an infected heart valve. In this case the embolus may contain bacteria from the infection that can cause an abscess at the site of embolism. Clots can also develop within a heart chamber if the heart becomes badly damaged, for example by a heart attack.
- **Air** A bubble of air can enter the circulation by accident during intravenous administration of fluid or drugs. Diving is also associated with air emboli. This condition is commonly known as the bends and is usually brought on by rising to the surface too quickly and by over-inflation of the lungs.
- **Amniotic fluid** This rare cause of embolism occurs during pregnancy. Under extreme circumstances, the fluid surrounding the baby may enter the veins in the pelvis.
- **Other materials** Fragments of tumors, fat, and cholesterol may also lead to embolism.

What are the symptoms?

The almost universal symptoms of embolism are pain and loss of function. An embolism in the leg, for instance, is associated with severe pain in the limb and loss of sensation. If a lung is affected, the person will experience chest pain and breathlessness. Kidney and intestinal embolism cause pain in the affected area. The only area that is not associated with pain when affected is the brain. Embolism in the brain causes a stroke, and the symptoms reflect the loss of function in the affected area.

How is it diagnosed?

For the most part, the diagnosis is usually suspected from the symptoms and a physical examination. Investigations are directed toward finding out the exact location of the blockage. Although computed tomography scanning, ultrasound (p. 109), and other imaging techniques may confirm the diagnosis, contrast X-rays of the affected arteries (angiography) may be needed (p. 109).

What are the treatment options?

The most important aspect of treatment is to reestablish the blood supply to the affected area before the tissue is irreversibly damaged. If the embolism is caused by a blood clot, doctors will probably prescribe "clot-busting" drugs (p. 118) and anticoagulants (p. 115) such as heparin and coumadin to dissolve the clot and prevent more clots from occurring. Balloon angioplasty (p. 119) can be carried out in the leg to clear some blockages. In certain cases—for example in pulmonary, kidney, intestinal, or limb embolism—emergency surgery may be necessary to remove the blockage and save the limb or organ involved. The bends are treated by a period inside a decompresssion chamber.

ENDOCARDITIS
Inflammation of the lining of the heart, caused by an infectious organism.

The heart muscle is lined on the inside by a thin layer called the endocardium, which coats the inner walls of the chambers (ventricles) of the heart and the valves themselves. If the endocardium becomes infected and inflamed, the resulting condition is known as endocarditis. If the areas lining the valves are affected, it's known as valvular endocarditis. Endocarditis is most frequently caused by two common bacteria, streptococci and staphylococci, so the condition is often referred to as bacterial endocarditis. It is estimated that every year in the United States about 6 people per 100,000 suffer from endocarditis.

Safety at the dentist

HELP YOUR DENTIST TO HELP YOU

If you are aware that a problem exists with one or more of your heart valves—for example if you have had a replacement valve—you are more at risk of contracting bacterial endocarditis from a visit to the dentist. This is because microorganisms, if disturbed, can enter the bloodstream from the mouth and travel to the heart. If necessary, you will be prescribed a single dose of an antibiotic to prevent any bacteria settling on the abnormal valve.

• *Always tell your dentist if you know of an existing problem with any of your heart valves.*

• *Inform the dentist if you are allergic to any antibiotics.*

What are the causes?
Endocarditis is caused by infectious organisms, such as bacteria, viruses, or fungi, which travel to the heart in the bloodstream from another part of the body. Those at risk of endocarditis are people who already have damaged areas in the heart's lining in which bacteria can nestle and begin to grow, for example people with congenital heart disease, with existing valve disease, or with artificial replacement valves. People who abuse intravenous drugs are also prone to endocarditis, because bacteria can be introduced into the bloodstream through dirty needles.

In endocarditis, a small plug of fibrin and platelets is deposited on a damaged area on the surface of the endocardium. When bacteria enter this plug, they multiply, resulting in a mass of cauliflower-like material commonly known as "vegetation," which forms a barrier around the bacteria. This mass gradually increases in size and can damage or obstruct a valve, impairing the heart's performance. It is not uncommon for a fragment of vegetation to become dislodged and travel in the bloodstream to the brain or the limbs, where it can become lodged in an artery and cut off the blood supply.

What are the symptoms?
The symptoms of endocarditis are very similar to those of a flu-like illness and may be mild at first. A person will probably experience one or more of the following:
• Weight loss
• Night sweats and a low-grade fever
• Pain in the joints
• Backache
• Tiredness
• Breathlessness
More serious symptoms develop if a fragment of vegetation, or embolus, breaks away from the valve. If the embolus travels to the brain, it can cause a stroke. If it blocks an artery in a limb, the blockage could result in severe pain and paralysis.

How is it diagnosed?
Doctors can diagnose many valve disorders by listening to the heart with a stethoscope (p. 100). If a person has endocarditis, an abnormal whooshing noise, known as a heart murmur, can be heard as the flow of blood becomes turbulent over the diseased valve. The diagnosis can sometimes be confirmed with an ultrasound scan of the heart—an echocardiogram (p. 106)—during which doctors may be able to visualize the vegetation.

What are the treatment options?

Treatment for endocarditis rests on successfully identifying the infecting organism because the doctor can then select the most appropriate antibiotic. The organisms are well protected in their microenvironment, and it is difficult for antibiotics to reach them. Treatment, therefore, needs to be administered intravenously for about four to six weeks. In approximately one-third of all cases, despite antibiotic therapy, surgery is required to remove the vegetation and, in valvular endocarditis, replace the damaged valve.

What is the outlook?

Most people who have valvular endocarditis are successfully treated. However, endocarditis of any kind can be fatal, especially if complications such as heart failure or stroke have occurred or if the infection has developed on an artificial valve.

GANGRENE
Tissue death because of a loss of blood supply and infection.

Healing of damaged areas of tissue can take place only if there is an abundant blood supply bringing nutrients and materials for the repair process. If this blood supply is lost, either from arterial disease or from death of the arteries within the damaged area, the body cannot carry out repairs, and the tissue finally dies and becomes gangrenous.

What are the causes?

The two main causes of gangrene are loss of the blood supply to the tissues, and infection. If the blood supply to part of the body is completely cut off, gangrene of the affected part will develop within hours if the blood supply is not restored. Trauma that severs arteries completely, an arterial embolism to the leg, or severe peripheral vascular disease can all precipitate gangrene.

Some bacteria also produce gas, which collects within the dead tissue—a condition known as gas gangrene.

Gangrene caused by infection develops when particular bacteria enter the skin at a site of injury, and toxic chemicals produced by the bacteria kill the surrounding cells. The bacteria multiply at a great rate as they feed off the dead cells and nutrients in the body so that the infection spreads rapidly. As a result, a minor area of damage can develop into a major life-threatening condition within hours of the initial infection.

What are the symptoms?

Whatever the cause of gangrene, the sufferer will experience severe pain in the affected area. Where an artery has been suddenly blocked or severed, the area starved of blood will also change color. Life-threatening secondary infection of the area can spread to affect the whole body. In some cases, for example in long-standing severe peripheral vascular disease, the changes are gradual, with a worsening of pain and a deterioration in the tissues of the extremities.

If infection is present, the individual becomes severely unwell within hours. The affected area initially looks pale, then becomes red and finally turns blackish green. Pockets of gas accumulating in the tissues may be felt with gentle pressure over the area.

How is it diagnosed?

Doctors will quickly diagnose gangrene from the characteristic appearance of the skin. If infection is suspected, samples of blood and fluid from the affected area are taken and examined microscopically for bacteria.

What are the treatment options?

Treatment for gangrene should begin immediately, so that as much tissue as possible is saved. If gangrene develops following an arterial injury or blockage, little can be done to restore the dead tissue, and amputation of the dead part of the affected limb is necessary. Long-standing peripheral vascular disease associated with small areas of gangrene may improve if the narrowed arteries are widened with angioplasty (p. 120). Nevertheless, if large areas of the limb become gangrenous, amputation may also be required.

Gangrene caused by infection is treated with injections of powerful antibiotics. Surgical removal of all dead and infected tissue is paramount and would usually be performed as an emergency operation.

HEART ATTACK
A reduction in the blood supply to the heart muscle leading to irreversible damage, also known as a myocardial infarction.

There is no doubt that having a heart attack is a frightening experience. Not only that, but the event happens more frequently than we would like to think—Many of us have a family member or friend who has suffered a heart attack. Most people survive an attack (about 60 percent), however, and, after a period of recovery, return to normal life.

What are the causes?

Like any other organ in the body, the heart needs its own supply of oxygenated blood to function. If one of the coronary arteries that transport this blood becomes blocked, the muscle tissue it supplies becomes starved of oxygen and will die within hours unless the blood supply is reestablished. A heart attack is usually caused by the development of a blood clot in one of the coronary arteries. The reason for this is the existence of fatty plaques called atheroma on the lining of the blood vessel wall. Sometimes, an atherosclerotic plaque becomes disrupted and exposes its contents to the bloodstream. This triggers a chain of events resulting in the accumulation of blood clot over the surface of the plaque, which can completely obstruct the flow of blood.

Heart attacks occur more frequently at certain times of the year, week, or day. The incidence peaks between 6:00 A.M. and 12:00 noon, at the start of the work week, and in the winter months (in temperate climates).

There are a number of risk factors that contribute to the development of atheroma:

- Smoking
- High blood cholesterol levels
- Obesity
- High blood pressure
- Diabetes mellitus
- A family history of coronary artery disease
- Male gender
- Increasing age

What are the symptoms?

It is important to emphasize that individual heart attacks can be experienced in many different ways, and even if an episode of chest pain does not have all the classic earmarks, it should still be taken seriously and medical advice should be sought promptly. In the elderly, for example, a heart attack may occur in the absence of all the symptoms listed below, with perhaps confusion being the only abnormality. As a guide, however, the following symptoms are very common during a heart attack:

- **Chest pain** Also known as angina, chest pain is frequently experienced during a heart attack. It usually comes on suddenly and grows in intensity over a matter of minutes. The pain is often described as "crushing" by those who have experienced it, and it can radiate down both arms and up into the jaw and throat.
- **Shortness of breath** In some people, especially the elderly, the only symptom of a heart attack is breathlessness, caused by an inability of the heart to pump properly so that excess fluid accumulates in the lungs.
- **Sweating** This symptom is often described as "breaking out in a cold sweat" because although perspiring profusely, the person may have cold hands and feet.
- **Nausea** About half of all people having a heart attack feel very sick to their stomachs during the early stages.
- **Palpitations** This awareness of the heart beating in the chest is caused by an increase in the heart rate.
- **Dizziness** A dizzy feeling may be followed by loss of consciousness. These symptoms are usually the result of an abnormal heartbeat.

Some people also experience a sudden urge to move their bowels, general weakness, and a feeling of impending death.

How is it diagnosed?

Often, the symptoms are a clear indication of the diagnosis. Doctors can be fairly sure that a person is having a heart attack simply from the medical history and an examination (p. 98). On the patient's arrival at the hospital, an electrocardiogram (p. 103) is carried out immediately to monitor heart electrical activity, and it often reveals the diagnosis instantly. Doctors will do blood tests (p. 102) to measure the levels of particular enzymes that rise when heart muscle is damaged. In some cases, angiography (p. 109) may be done with a view to reopening the blocked artery (angioplasty).

Can I have a heart attack with no symptoms?

Research suggests that 25 percent of heart attacks may go unrecognized and are only discovered later when a routine ECG is carried out. In half of these cases, the individual may recall a few suggestive symptoms following some prompting from the doctor. So-called silent heart attacks are more common among people with diabetes, high blood pressure, or angina. The mechanism is unclear, but doctors believe it to be related to higher pain thresholds and an abnormality of the cardiac nervous system, which is involved in relaying the painful stimulus to the brain. Patients who have suffered silent heart attacks should be treated in a similar way to those who have suffered a "symptomatic" heart attack, with particular attention to risk factors and lifestyle changes.

ASK THE EXPERT

143

What are the treatment options?

A person who has had a heart attack will probably be admitted to a coronary care unit, where bed rest and continual monitoring of heart rhythm are essential over the initial 48 hours. Treatment varies depending on the extent of damage to the heart, but the primary aims of therapy are to relieve pain and breathlessness and restore blood flow through the blocked coronary artery as soon as possible. This can be achieved more easily soon after the onset of chest pain—If treatment is started within the first few hours of symptoms developing, the risk of a heart attack being fatal is reduced by about 20 to 30 percent.

Doctors will immediately prescribe strong intravenous painkillers (morphine) and oxygen, as well as a dose of aspirin to thin the blood and an intravenous infusion of a drug that breaks down the blood clot—This drug is far more effective if given within the first few hours after a heart attack. Additional medications may also be given to help prevent subsequent heart attacks; these include beta-blockers, more aspirin, and cholesterol-lowering drugs.

Once a person is stable and the pain has lessened, there are several options. In some cases, the artery can be re-opened with a procedure called coronary angioplasty (p. 120). People who have severe narrowing of more than one artery may need surgery—coronary artery bypass grafting (p. 124)—to relieve the blockage.

What is the outlook?

Thanks to increased awareness of lifestyle issues, the rate of death following a heart attack is falling. In Europe, 75 to 80 percent of individuals suffering a heart attack are still alive a year later. It is difficult to predict how many will go on to have another attack, but preventative treatment is given to all high-risk individuals.

HEART FAILURE

An inability of the heart to pump blood effectively around the body.

When a person has heart failure, it doesn't mean that the heart has completely stopped working, but that it has become less efficient and is unable to keep up with all the body's demands for a healthy supply of oxygen-rich blood. The extent of heart failure varies from person to person: Some individuals have no symptoms at all and are able to live normal lives, whereas others are severely affected and even housebound because of their restricted mobility.

What are the causes?

Anything that affects the heart's ability to beat effectively can cause heart failure. Almost two-thirds of heart failure cases are due to damaged heart muscle caused by severe coronary artery disease—narrowing of the arteries that supply the heart muscle with oxygen-rich blood—especially following a heart attack. High blood pressure is the second most common cause of heart failure; years of pumping against high pressure puts damaging strain on the muscle tissue. Heart failure can also result from either leaking or tight heart valves.

Less frequently, heart failure results from injury caused by toxins, such as alcohol or recreational drugs, circulating in the bloodstream. Some viral infections can also inflict damage on the heart muscle, for example the Coxsackie virus, which usually causes only a minor flu-like illness. Rarely, heart failure can result from diseases occurring elsewhere in the body, such as thyroid disease and some types of arthritis. In very rare cases heart failure can be caused by vitamin and mineral deficiencies.

What are the symptoms?

For many people, heart failure is symptomless, especially in the early stages of the condition. Generally, however, the symptoms reflect the extent and location of damage in the heart. For example, failure of the left ventricle (the pumping chamber) typically causes problems with breathing as fluid accumulates in the lungs—a condition known as pulmonary edema. Breathing difficulties become worse during exertion, when the body's oxygen requirements increase, or when lying flat because the left ventricle cannot cope with the increased rate of blood returning to the heart. Occasionally, a person may wake in the early hours of the morning gasping for breath, with a feeling of suffocation, wheezing, or tightness in the chest. In such cases urgent medical treatment should be sought.

Other symptoms reflect the reduced blood supply to various organs of the body; these are as follows:
- Muscle weakness
- Loss of appetite
- Cold hands and feet
- Lightheadedness or confusion

If the ventricle in the right side of the heart is pumping inadequately, excess fluid accumulates in the body's tissues, most obviously in the feet and legs.

Heart failure is afflicting increasing numbers of people each year in the developed world. Overall, in the United States, 1 percent of people aged 50, but 5 percent of people aged 75, are affected.

In most cases of heart failure both of the ventricles are damaged and sufferers experience a combination of the symptoms of right and left ventricular failure.

How is it diagnosed?

The doctor will usually be able to make a diagnosis of heart failure from the symptoms and a physical examination (p. 98). Often, even the extent of heart damage and the cause can be determined at the initial consultation. The doctor will, however, carry out tests to confirm the diagnosis, including the following:

- Echocardiogram This ultrasound scan of the heart (p. 106) identifies any underlying heart disorders.
- Electrocardiogram The doctor may look at tracings of the heart's electrical activity (p. 103).
- Nuclear scans These specialized scans (p. 108) highlight abnormalities and help to define the blood supply to the heart muscle.
- Coronary angiograms If coronary artery disease is suspected, doctors may carry out angiograms (p. 109).

An exciting development in recent years has been the identification of a substance—natriuretic peptide—produced by the heart when it is failing. In the future, this may lead to a simple blood test to diagnose heart failure.

What are the treatment options?

The first step the doctor will take is to treat the cause of the heart failure. Evidence suggests that the rate of progression of heart failure can be slowed by controlling blood pressure, replacing damaged heart valves, and, in some cases, by opening narrowed coronary arteries by angioplasty (p. 120) or surgery.

Drug therapy can be helpful in controlling the symptoms of heart failure. Diuretic drugs encourage the kidneys to get rid of the excess fluid that accumulates, particularly in the lower legs and the lungs. For reasons that remain unclear, one particular diuretic called spironolactone has recently been shown to be exceptionally useful in slowing the rate at which heart failure progresses. Over the past 10 to 15 years, angiotensin converting enzyme (ACE) inhibitors have revolutionized the treatment of heart failure (p. 114). Numerous research studies have shown that these drugs, which lower blood pressure and in some cases prevent further heart muscle damage, can greatly reduce the heart's workload. More recently, evidence has emerged showing that beta-blockers, which slow the heart rate and force of contraction, can increase survival and relieve symptoms of heart failure.

What is the outlook?

Heart failure is a progressive disease that if left untreated is eventually fatal. However, the drug treatments currently available are powerful and have been shown to improve the length and quality of life for patients with heart failure.

HEART INFECTIONS

See Endocarditis, p. 141, Myocarditis, p. 149, Pericarditis, p. 149.

HEART VALVE DISEASE

Conditions in which heart valves become stiff and/or narrowed, or fail to close properly, thereby affecting the blood flow within the heart.

The openings to the heart's four chambers are controlled by one-way valves, which ensure that the 9500 quarts of blood pumped through the heart each day flows in one direction only. With all this work, the valves are bound to suffer wear and tear, and many elderly people have a degree of valve incompetence even though it may be asymptomatic. In some people, however, one (or more) of the heart valves become diseased or damaged and cause symptoms. The two valves most frequently affected are the aortic valve, which separates the left ventricle from the main artery of the body—the aorta—and the mitral valve, which divides the two left chambers.

What are the causes?

There are two ways in which heart valves become problematic: When a valve becomes narrow or stiff, it can fail to open properly, a condition known as stenosis; if the valve is unable to close completely, blood tends to flow backward—regurgitation—and the valve is said to be incompetent. Either of these situations can disrupt the flow of blood and adversely affect the structure of the heart. In the past, the most common cause of a damaged heart valve was rheumatic fever, a condition that is now rarely encountered. These days, doctors are more likely to diagnose the following causes.

- Bacterial endocarditis Organisms travel to the heart in the bloodstream and infect one or more valves.
- Calcium deposits These build up on the aortic valve, causing narrowing—a condition called aortic stenosis.
- Coronary artery disease or heart attack The damage sustained by the heart can extend to the muscles that

support the valves so that they are unable to close properly, causing a condition known as regurgitation.

• **Congenital abnormalities** Some babies are born with an existing defect, typically a misshapen aortic or bicuspid valve, or very rarely a narrowed mitral valve.

What are the symptoms?

Most valve abnormalities that progress gradually cause no symptoms until very late in their development, and the problem is picked up only at a routine checkup. If nothing is done, then in the long term the heart may fail to cope with its increased workload and heart failure can develop. Abnormal valves are also vulnerable to infection, which can erode them rapidly and lead to a medical emergency.

How is it diagnosed?

A good clinical examination will reveal the nature and likely severity of a heart valve problem. Echocardiography (p. 106)—ultrasound of the heart—is now the key investigative technique to confirm the diagnosis; it also allows the progress of the abnormality and its effect on heart function to be assessed over long-term follow-up. The transesophageal approach for echocardiography is sometimes necessary to assess the mitral valve accurately.

What are the treatment options?

People with heart valve disease are usually carefully monitored in a doctor's office and have regular echocardiograms. The aim is usually to delay surgery for as long as possible, without allowing permanent damage to develop. Patients are advised to have antibiotic cover prior to dental procedures, which can trigger the release of bacteria into the bloodstream for a brief period and could result in bacterial endocarditis.

Ultimately, valve-replacement surgery (p. 129) may be necessary. In these operations, the surgeon usually completely removes the diseased valve and substitutes a mechanical or biological tissue valve for it. In some cases, however, the mitral valve can be stretched open if it is narrowed or repaired if it is leaky.

What is the outlook?

People with heart valve disease usually make a good recovery following valve replacement surgery, although those fitted with mechanical valves require lifelong treatment with anticoagulant drugs (p. 115) to thin the blood and reduce the risk of blood clots. They will also require antibiotic cover for dental procedures. Biological

tissue valves may become chalky and progressively fail over the years, so such valves are generally reserved for the elderly in whom the risk of blood thinning is a more important consideration.

HYPERTENSION

Persistently high blood pressure, which if left untreated may cause damage to the body's organs.

High blood pressure is a very common problem in the United States and is a major risk factor for cardiovascular disease, contributing to the high incidence of heart disease and stroke. The problem with hypertension is that it is virtually symptomless until the condition begins to cause damage in other parts of the body. Hence, it is often only diagnosed during a routine examination.

What is the cause?

The majority of people with persistently high blood pressure have what is termed essential hypertension. This means that there is no single identifiable cause for the problem. Essential hypertension is thought to reflect the interaction of an individual's genetic make-up with congenital and environmental factors such as low birth weight, high dietary salt with low fruit and vegetable intake, sedentary lifestyle, obesity, excess alcohol consumption, and social status. In addition, blood pressure naturally rises with age in Western communities.

High blood pressure is associated with excessive consumption of licorice-based products.

In a small percentage of people, the elevation of their blood pressure occurs as a result of disease of the kidneys or of the adrenal, thyroid, or pituitary glands. Long-term use of steroid drugs is also associated with hypertension.

What are the symptoms?

Hypertension rarely causes symptoms—These are more likely to arise from associated diseases, such as coronary artery disease, peripheral vascular disease, aortic aneurysm, or stroke. Occasionally, people may experience headaches and nosebleeds that are thought to be associated with hypertension. Long-term hypertension may eventually lead to thickening of the muscle of the heart, which can cause the symptoms of heart failure. Rarely, hypertension can cause sudden and severe damage, for example a burst aortic aneurysm, brain hemorrhage, or, during pregnancy, preeclampsia or eclampsia.

How is it diagnosed?

Most people discover that their blood pressure is high when they see their doctor for some other reason. Sometimes it is discovered at the time of a complication or associated disease. Except in the case of the emergencies discussed earlier, hypertension can only be diagnosed if several readings taken on different days show that the blood pressure is greater than 140/90 millimeters of mercury.

The doctor will also examine the person's eyes and test a sample of urine, since hypertension may cause damage to the retina at the back of the eye and the kidneys. Tests are usually performed to check for an underlying cause. Initially, these involve blood tests (p. 102), chest X-ray (p. 105) and electrocardiogram (p. 103). If any of these tests show abnormalities, further tests will be required.

What are the treatment options?

The aims of treatment of essential hypertension are to prevent blood pressure from becoming even higher and to avoid the development of heart disease. It should form part of a wider approach in which other risk factors such as high cholesterol and smoking are addressed. Some people at high risk of cardiovascular disease may benefit from daily aspirin once the blood pressure is well controlled.

There are two ways in which blood pressure can be lowered in essential hypertension: lifestyle measures and drug treatment. All people with hypertension should aim to adopt a healthy lifestyle. Specific changes that help to lower blood pressure include reduction in dietary salt, with increased fruit and vegetable intake, appropriate weight loss, sensible exercise, and moderation of alcohol intake.

Many people with mild hypertension will require a regular blood pressure check to make sure it remains within acceptable limits. People with blood pressure consistently higher than 140/90 will probably need drug therapy (p. 113), as will people who have signs of complications from the hypertension. The major problem with drugs for hypertension is that they can produce side effects ranging from drowsiness to impotence. Because hypertension is largely asymptomatic, it can be difficult for people to accept medication-related symptoms, especially because therapy will need to be continued for several years, if not for life. However, the number of drugs available to treat hypertension is large and continuing to grow, so it is usually possible to find a regime that is well tolerated.

In people with hypertension related to another condition, treatment will be directed at correcting the cause, although antihypertensive medication may still be needed.

How can it be prevented or minimized?

Living a healthy lifestyle will not only help to reduce the likelihood of developing essential hypertension but will also reduce the progression of the disease over time and the length of time medication will be required to control the blood pressure.

HYPOTENSION

A blood pressure level that is abnormally low for a particular individual.

Many healthy people have blood pressure that is lower than the "average." This is not harmful and just reflects that person's individual characteristics. For example, people who are very fit normally have low blood pressure. Blood pressure varies enormously with activity and is usually lowest in the middle of the night when we are asleep. Hypotension, however, is an abnormally low pressure— lower than the "normal" range of pressure for an individual.

What are the causes?

There are five main reasons for hypotension.

- **Decreased blood volume** The amount of blood in the circulation can drop due to blood loss, for example, or dehydration. When this happens, the heart beats harder and faster to maintain the pressure in the system, but eventually, if the volume is not replaced, these compensatory mechanisms fail and blood pressure falls.

Does my temper influence my blood pressure?

Anger does cause physiological changes in the body. When we lose our temper, a surge of hormones— notably epinephrine and norepinephrine—is released from the adrenal glands into the bloodstream. One of the effects of these hormones is to cause constriction of the blood vessels throughout the body as part of the natural "fight-or-flight" mechanism. With this narrowing of the arteries, there is an increase in resistance to the flow of blood, so the pressure goes up.

In fact, several research studies back this up, showing that people who lose their temper easily are at greater risk of developing hypertension and heart disease.

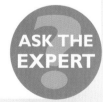

ASK THE EXPERT

- **Heart failure** If the heart fails to pump properly, for example after a heart attack, it is unable to maintain the pressure in the circulation, and blood pressure drops.
- **Dilation of the blood vessels** Some illnesses, many of them infections, can cause the blood vessels to widen. The volume of blood within the circulation may not be able to increase quickly enough to fill the increased space and, if the heart cannot compensate, blood pressure falls.
- **Postural hypotension** Some people have a tendency to faint if they have to stand for long periods, especially in hot weather. In such situations, there is a temporary loss of control of blood pressure and heart rate, and both fall dramatically, causing a loss of consciousness.
- **Drugs** Some medications, particularly those used to treat high blood pressure, can cause hypotension.

What are the symptoms?
Mild hypotension often causes no symptoms at all. As blood pressure falls, people may notice that they feel

Tall, lean people are more likely to have low blood pressure and have a greater tendency to faint.

lightheaded when they stand up and may have to reach for support to stop themselves from falling. If the blood pressure remains low, eventually the sensation of lightheadedness may persist continuously. Fainting episodes may occur, and people frequently feel sick and may vomit. When very severe, the level of consciousness starts to decrease; eventually, at a critically low blood pressure, coma ensues.

How is it diagnosed?
A diagnosis of hypotension is made when blood pressure readings are lower than expected, compared with previous values. The doctor may confirm this by taking measurements with the patient lying down and standing up—A person with hypotension will show a significant drop in pressure when standing. Unless obvious, further investigations to uncover the cause are usually necessary.

What are the treatment options?
The treatment options vary enormously according to the cause of hypotension, but treating the cause usually returns the blood pressure to normal; for example, giving fluid in cases of dehydration, a blood transfusion after a hemorrhage, or antibiotics to treat an infection. Hypotension with no known cause is rare and is usually difficult to treat. If the symptoms are persistent, however, doctors may prescribe drugs in the short term to constrict the blood vessels and increase blood pressure.

KAWASAKI'S DISEASE
A rare condition affecting children, in which arteries throughout the body become inflamed.

Experts do not fully understand why the arteries become inflamed in this disease, but some families appear to be at greater risk, especially those of Japanese descent. Kawasaki's disease predominantly affects children under the age of five, although there have been rare reports of the disease in people as old as 34.

In about 10 percent of cases, the disease attacks the heart, causing inflammation and damage to the heart muscle. The arteries supplying the heart can become weakened, and aneurysms—bulges in the artery walls—can develop. Although these aneurysms can burst, the main risk is clot formation in the affected artery, blocking it and causing a heart attack.

What are the symptoms?
The disease usually starts with flu-like symptoms of fever, tiredness, aching joints, and feeling unwell. The glands in the neck are often enlarged and tender. After a day or two, the following symptoms appear one after the other:
- A rash on the trunk
- A sore mouth and eyes
- Red and swollen palms and soles

In the majority of cases, the disease starts to subside at this point, with complete recovery usually occurring within 2 to 12 weeks. Alternatively, at this time the heart can begin to be affected, producing symptoms of breathlessness, chest pain, or palpitations.

How is it diagnosed?
The diagnosis of Kawasaki's disease is difficult and is based upon the recognition of the characteristic symptoms. Blood tests (p. 102) are largely unhelpful in confirming the disease, although they are essential to exclude other illnesses that may present similar symptoms. Echocardiography (p. 106) is performed in all cases at about the fifth week, and coronary angiography (p. 109) may be done if doctors suspect coronary artery aneurysms.

What are the treatment options?
If aspirin is given early on, it has been shown to reduce the risk of heart complications. More recently, doctors have treated children with injections of specific proteins, called immunoglobulins, that are involved in the body's defense system and that further reduce this risk.

What is the outlook?

The majority of children with Kawasaki's disease recover completely and, in time, most coronary artery aneurysms heal. Occasionally the condition can be fatal, however, because of heart failure resulting from inflammation of the heart muscle or because of a ruptured aneurysm.

MYOCARDIAL INFARCTION
See Heart attack, p. 142 to 144.

MYOCARDITIS
A rare condition involving inflammation of the heart muscle, usually caused by infection.

The muscle of the heart, the myocardium, can become inflamed as a result of infection, a rare condition known as myocarditis. The inflammation is usually a complication of an infection with a virus, bacteria, parasite, or fungus—in the Western world, usually the virus Coxsackie Type B. The initial infection causes particular proteins to be released from the heart muscle cells; the body's defense system does not recognize these proteins and mistakenly attacks the heart muscle, contributing further to the inflammation.

What are the symptoms?

There is often a period of weeks between the initial infection and the development of myocarditis, when symptoms may include the following:
- Chest discomfort (often confused with angina)
- Fatigue
- Breathlessness and palpitations

Myocarditis often is accompanied by pericarditis (see right), an inflammation of the heart's outer membrane. Rarely, the damage to the heart muscle is more serious and, over a period of time, heart failure can develop.

How is it diagnosed?

Doctors may suspect myocarditis from the symptoms, especially if these occur in conjunction with another infectious illness. Often, however, by the time symptoms appear, the infectious organism is difficult to detect, although doctors may locate the organism in blood, stool, or throat swabs. An ultrasound scan of the heart, an echocardiogram (p. 106), may detect a damaged heart. In rare instances, a tiny sample of tissue may be taken from the heart muscle for examination.

What are the treatment options?

The majority of cases of myocarditis are mild, and people usually recover fully after two weeks of rest. If the infection is caused by an organism other than a virus, then antibiotics will be given. If heart failure develops, doctors will treat the symptoms accordingly.

PERICARDITIS
An inflammation of the pericardium, the protective membrane that envelops the heart.

The pericardium is a stiff, flask-shaped sac that helps prevent excessive motion of the heart and provides a barrier to infection from surrounding organs. There are two layers to the pericardium, separated from each other by a small amount of fluid, so there's no friction. Inflammation of this outer layer is called pericarditis and is often, but not always, caused by infection from viruses, bacteria (including tuberculosis), and fungi. Pericarditis is also associated with other conditions, such as arthritis and kidney failure. In developed countries, tuberculous pericarditis has declined as a result of effective vaccination, but tuberculosis still remains the major cause of pericarditis in the developing world.

What are the symptoms?

The main symptom of pericarditis is pain in the chest, neck, shoulder, or upper abdomen. Typically the pain is aggravated by breathing in, coughing, and lying flat and relieved by sitting forward. If the pericarditis is secondary to another infection in the body, the symptoms of that infection will also be present. A chest infection, for example, may cause breathlessness.

Some people with pericarditis can "feel" the membranes rubbing together in their chest.

Sometimes, the fluid between the membranes temporarily increases in volume because of the inflammation, a condition known as a pericardial effusion. If the fluid collection is large enough, it can exert pressure on the heart and affect its function—a potentially life-threatening situation called cardiac tamponade

If the inflammation persists for a long time, the pericardium may become thickened and scarred and prevent the heart from beating properly—a rare but serious condition known as constrictive pericarditis. In all these instances, a person may experience the symptoms of heart failure, such as breathlessness and swelling of the tissues.

How is it diagnosed?

The easiest way to diagnose pericarditis is to listen to the heart through a stethoscope (p. 100). A scratching sound, known as a pericardial rub, can frequently be heard; it is thought to be the sound of friction between the roughened pericardial layers. The doctor may arrange for an electrocardiogram (p. 103) to monitor the heart's electrical activity and blood tests (p. 102) to indicate the presence of infection. Excess fluid accumulation around the heart can usually be seen on an echocardiogram (p. 106). The thickened pericardium often shows up on a chest X-ray (p. 105). Abnormal thickening of the pericardium can also be visualized with high-resolution scanning techniques such as magnetic resonance imaging (p. 108).

What are the treatment options?

The doctor will probably treat the inflammation and pain with nonsteroidal antiinflammatory drugs and recommend rest during the course of the illness. If the inflammation is caused by an infectious organism, then that organism will be treated with appropriate drugs, such as antibiotics. If excess fluid has accumulated in the pericardial sac, the doctor will need to remove the fluid with a needle and syringe under local anesthetic. If constrictive pericarditis develops, surgery may be necessary to remove the pericardium completely.

What is the outlook?

The outlook for people with pericarditis is variable and depends on the cause of the inflammation. Viral pericarditis has the best outlook and usually clears up within a week. Bacterial pericarditis is more serious, however, so the recovery time is normally longer, especially if surgery to remove the pericardium is involved.

PERIPHERAL VASCULAR DISEASE

In this condition, a build-up of fatty deposits in blood vessels leads to impaired blood supply to the legs.

Arteries are a vital network of blood vessels, delivering oxygen- and nutrient-rich blood to tissues throughout the body. Any blockage or narrowing that develops in the arteries impedes the flow of blood and deprives the tissues of vital life support. This is exactly what happens in peripheral vascular disease: The arteries that supply the limbs with blood become clogged up by fatty deposits— a condition known as atherosclerosis.

What is the cause?

Atherosclerosis in the peripheral arteries develops for the same reasons that it does in the coronary arteries of the heart. Excess fats circulating in the blood stick to areas of the lining of arteries that are roughened or slightly damaged, causing a narrowing of the vessel and sometimes even a complete blockage. (See pages 94 to 95 for the risk factors for atherosclerosis.)

Amazingly, if an artery is blocked, the body organizes an alternative route by widening nearby smaller arteries.

What are the symptoms?

The most significant symptom of peripheral vascular disease is intermittent claudication—a cramp-like pain in the calves, thighs, and/or buttocks that occurs because the muscles are deprived of oxygen. Usually, people notice the pain during exertion, such as walking up a hill or climbing flights of stairs, and the pain is rapidly relieved when they rest. As the disease becomes worse and the arteries progressively narrow, pain develops with less and less exertion until, eventually, it is present even at rest.

In very severe cases, ulcers may develop on the toes as the tissue dies due to lack of oxygen, and occasionally gangrene starts to develop in areas where the blood supply is insufficient to keep the muscle and skin alive.

How is it diagnosed?

Progressive tests are carried out to diagnose the extent and location of the narrowings.

- **Physical examination of the legs** Just as we have an arterial pulse at the wrist, we have pulses in our legs (p. 100). These become weak or disappear altogether in people with peripheral arterial disease.
- **Doppler studies** This ultrasound scanning technique (p. 109) is used on the arteries of the legs to show blood flow within the arteries.
- **Angiography** Injection of a radiopaque dye into the arteries of the legs allows doctors to obtain clear X-ray images of the blood supply (p. 109).

What are the treatment options?

The doctor will make a decision about treatment based on how badly the arteries are narrowed and how much pain the person is experiencing. Aspirin and cholesterol-lowering therapy may be prescribed—These measures will help to prevent further narrowing in the leg arteries as well as protecting the rest of the circulation; often coronary, cerebral, and renal vessels are also affected. For many people with mild symptoms, no other specific treatment is required. Unlike cases of narrowing of the heart arteries, exercise should be encouraged; it will not cause any harm and may stimulate the widening of other arteries to effectively bypass any arterial blockages. Exercise activity should be continued as long as the pain is bearable. Although many people will eventually have to rest, some find that the pain gets less as they continue. Doctors describe this as "walking through the pain."

If pain begins to limit activity severely, and if the main arteries of the legs have become diseased, more aggressive treatment may be necessary. Angioplasty (p. 120) can be performed to dilate the narrowed areas in the arteries. If the disease is too severe to be tackled by this approach, bypass surgery (p. 124) may need to be performed on one or both legs. If the disease is very severe, especially if gangrene is evident, amputation of part of the affected limb may need to be considered.

RAYNAUD'S DISEASE/PHENOMENON

Excessive spasm in the arteries of the fingers or toes, particularly in cold weather.

Many people notice that their hands become almost painfully cold if they go outdoors on a frosty day without gloves, or even that their fingers turn blue. Although often blamed on "bad circulation," this usually has little to do with arterial disease, reflecting a normal response to the cold. The body conserves heat by rerouting blood from the extremities, where heat is easily lost, to the body's core.

In some people, however, exposure to cold precipitates an excessive contraction (spasm) of the muscle in the arterial wall, a condition called Raynaud's disease. This results in troublesome symptoms and occasionally, in the long term, damage to the fingers and toes.

What is the cause?

Raynaud's disease is most common in young women and is diagnosed when there is no other obvious cause for the symptoms. There are many diseases and a few drugs that can precipitate symptoms identical to those of Raynaud's disease, when the term *Raynaud's phenomenon* is used. In either case, doctors do not fully understand the cause.

What are the symptoms?

Attacks may last minutes or hours and are commonly precipitated by exposure of the hands or feet to cold, which may not necessarily be severe, or occasionally by stress,

emotional upset, or exercise. The condition usually affects both hands and is characterised by the following:

- A dramatic color change in the affected fingers and toes, which appear white or dark purple. There may be a well-defined border to the affected area, with normal colour skin on the other side.
- A feeling of "pins and needles," although the fingers are not usually painful.
- When warming the hands, the affected areas become red before returning to normal.

In some people with long-standing severe Raynaud's disease/phenomenon, damage to the fingers and toes may occur. Typically, the tips of the fingers and toes become narrowed with skin that is smooth, shiny, and tight. Small painful breaks in the skin, or ulcers, may also form.

How is it diagnosed?

The doctor will probably suspect Raynaud's from the symptoms, which are quite specific. The challenge is to distinguish Raynaud's disease from Raynaud's phenomenon, a distinction that is more easily made if there are additional symptoms. If Raynaud's phenomenon is suspected, investigations will be needed to identify the underlying cause.

EXPERIENCING RAYNAUD'S DISEASE

Ever since I was a child, I have had poor circulation in my fingers and toes, which would quickly go blue if I wasn't wrapped up well enough.

One day I was out walking the dog without gloves, on a morning that turned out to be extremely cold. My hands started to tingle and I looked down to see that the tips of my fingers had gone white. They were quite numb and started turning purple. I actually started to worry I might have some sort of frostbite, and went straight to my doctor.

The doctor said I had Raynaud's disease and reassured me that I wasn't about to lose my fingers. She explained that in most cases like mine, treatment wasn't necessary, and I should simply wear gloves and warm footwear when outdoors and give up smoking. However, if the symptoms worsened, she said I should go back and see her again.

What are the treatment options?

Mild cases of Raynaud's disease can be managed simply by wearing thick gloves in cold weather. Smoking exacerbates the condition and so should be avoided. If symptoms are more troublesome, drugs to promote the relaxation of the arterial muscle can be used to reduce both the frequency and severity of attacks. In very severe cases, in which constant attacks threaten to cause tissue death, surgery to cut the nerves that control arterial contraction—known as a sympathectomy—may be necessary. In Raynaud's phenomenon, treatment is directed toward the underlying condition, although some of the measures discussed earlier may also be appropriate.

SHOCK

A life-threatening condition associated with critically reduced blood flow.

In medical terms, shock describes a state in which the blood supply to vital organs becomes inadequate and their function becomes impaired. If the blood supply is not restored quickly enough, permanent damage to the organs may occur. This severe condition can be fatal if treatment is not started quickly. There are two main types of shock: hypovolemic shock and cardiogenic shock.

- **Hypovolemic shock** If there is a fall in the volume of blood in the circulation, the amount pumped out by the heart with each contraction (the cardiac output) is reduced. In an effort to maintain an adequate blood flow to the body, the heart rate speeds up. If blood loss is severe, or is not treated, eventually the heart is unable to cope. The cardiac output becomes completely inadequate, and hypovolemic shock results.
- **Cardiogenic shock** This second major type of shock results mainly from diseases of the heart. As heart disease reduces the cardiac output, the body compensates by diverting blood from nonessential areas such as the limbs to essential organs such as the brain. If output continues to fall, however, even this diversion mechanism cannot maintain adequate blood supply to the organs.

What are the causes?

There are many causes of hypovolemic shock, including:

- Severe bleeding as a result of trauma, surgery, or a disorder such as an aortic aneurysm
- Loss of other body fluids through extensive skin burns, or perforation or infection of the gut

- Excessive loss of urine caused by diabetes or kidney disease
- Widening of the blood vessels (vasodilation) in the body so that even though the circulating blood volume is normal, it is not adequate to fill the increased capacity. This can happen when the vessels dramatically dilate in response to disease. A severe bacterial infection such as pneumonia is one cause of this and is a direct result of the actions of toxins and other chemicals released both by the bacteria and by the body's defense systems.
- Liver failure and the ingestion of some poisons
- Inadequate fluid intake, usually as a result of failing to replace a modest increase in fluid loss, as happens, for example, in diarrhea or profuse vomiting

Cardiogenic shock can sometimes result from severe damage to heart muscle following a heart attack. It can also be a complication of severe disease of the heart valves, abnormal heart rhythms, or compression of the heart by either a collection of fluid or blood or by a collapsed lung.

A pulmonary embolus—a clot in an artery supplying the lungs—sometimes causes shock if the blood flow through the lungs is severely reduced by the blockage.

What are the symptoms?

Confusion and drowsiness are common symptoms of shock, resulting from the reduced blood flow to the brain. When shock becomes more severe, the affected person usually loses consciousness. The hands and feet become cold and moist, with a bluish tinge, as the body tries to compensate for falling cardiac output by diverting blood from the limbs to the vital organs. If shock is caused by infection, fever and episodes of uncontrollable shivering are often present—In these cases the skin is warm and flushed.

How is it diagnosed?

Shock is a life-threatening condition, the symptoms of which are usually immediately obvious to the doctor. An abnormally low blood pressure together with evidence of reduced blood supply to vital organs—confusion, poor blood flow to the hands and feet, decreased urine output, rapid heartbeat, and breathing rate—all indicate a medical emergency. The underlying cause is often clear, but sometimes a person will need urgent further investigation.

What are the treatment options?

The doctor's priority in treating shock is to restore the blood supply to vital organs before permanent damage develops. Usually, medical treatment takes place in an intensive care unit, where specialist nursing care and

24-hour monitoring are available. If doctors suspect hypovolemic shock, prompt intravenous infusions of blood and other fluids are given into cannulae placed into veins in the arms and neck. If the response is not rapid, or cardiogenic shock is suspected, infusions of powerful drugs will be given to maintain blood pressure. In cases where the lungs are failing, or if the patient is unconscious, artificial ventilation will be needed for a period of time. If the kidneys have stopped working, dialysis may be necessary to carry out their functions until they recover.

Although maintaining the circulation and supporting lung function is the highest priority, treatment for the underlying cause will be started as early as possible. For example, if the patient has an infection, antibiotics can be started immediately. Further investigations and surgical procedures usually have to wait until the blood pressure has been stabilized.

TACHYCARDIA

A fast heart rate that may be a normal response to exercise or stress but may also be caused by an abnormal rhythm of the heartbeat.

The electrical impulses that stimulate the heart's contractions originate in an area called the sinoatrial node, also known as the "pacemaker." Each impulse travels through the heart in a set pattern—almost as though it were following a system of wiring—activating contraction of the chambers of the heart in the correct order. The speed at which these impulses fire, and at which the heart beats, is controlled by many factors, including nerve signals and hormones circulating in the blood. Tachycardia is said to occur when the heart beats faster than the accepted normal range of 60 to 90 beats per minute. It is perfectly normal for the heart to beat faster during exercise or stress. However, an unusually fast rate—a tachyarrhythmia—can be caused by an abnormality. In these instances, the heart may beat fast at inappropriate times, for example at night or when resting.

In some people, too much coffee or alcohol can precipitate a fast heart rate.

What are the causes?

A tachyarrhythmia can develop if the heart muscle is damaged or if there is faulty wiring, both of which affect the transmission of impulses within the heart. This can occur as a result of heart muscle or valve disease,

Describing palpitations

Remember that it is a normal bodily response to have a fast heartbeat when we exercise or become anxious. However, palpitations that occur at unusual times, for example when resting, or that are severe enough to wake you from sleep, are much more suspicious, especially if they are associated with chest pain, breathlessness, or feeling faint. If in doubt, talk to your doctor. Try to note the following:

- *When did the palpitations occur and what were you doing at the time?*

- *Is there any pattern to the attacks, or is there an obvious precipitating event?*

Learn to take your own pulse and record your heart rate in beats per minute when palpitations occur. If you are aware of any irregular heartbeat, can you tap in time with it, or does the rate seem to change from beat to beat?

congenital heart abnormalities, certain drugs, and thyroid problems. There are two main categories of tachyarrhythmia relating to the chambers of the heart that are involved:

- **Supraventricular tachycardias** These arise when the abnormality lies within or near the upper chambers—the atria. Fast electrical impulses cause the atria to contract at a rapid rate, and in a chaotic and disorganized fashion. When atrial activity is too chaotic, the atria cannot contract properly, a state known as atrial fibrillation, which is very common among elderly people. Some or all of the fast impulses generated within the atria are transmitted to the ventricle, which then also beats faster.

- **Ventricular tachycardia** This arrhythmia arises when an abnormality in the ventricles causes rapid contraction of these chambers. This is usually more serious than supraventricular tachycardias, since the ventricle may not be able to pump blood properly around the body, leading to shock. Ventricular tachycardia can eventually progress to cardiac arrest, either on its own or by precipitating ventricular fibrillation when the activity of the ventricles becomes completely disorganized. If not promptly treated, cardiac arrest is fatal.

What are the symptoms?

The severity of the symptoms depends upon the particular tachyarrhythmia concerned. The most common symptom associated with supraventricular tachyarrhythmias is palpitations, an awareness of the heart beating in the chest. This derives from the fast rate of ventricular contraction and is usually described as a fluttering sensation. It may be associated with shortness of breath, chest pain, or giddiness. Rarely, people may faint in response to this arrhythmia. In supraventricular tachycardia, the pattern of these symptoms may be intermittent or continuous . In the former, people may notice events that precipitate a bout of palpitations, such as drinking too much coffee or alcohol.

Although ventricular tachycardia may cause symptoms similar to those of supraventricular tachycardias, it is more likely to cause severe illness with loss of consciousness. Ventricular fibrillation always causes unconsciousness, which rapidly progresses to death if not treated promptly.

How is it diagnosed?

The doctor is often able to detect a tachycardia or tachyarrhythmia just by feeling the pulse. The abnormality is usually confirmed by electrocardiography—ECG—(p. 103) and often requires investigation by a cardiologist.

HAVING PALPITATIONS

I was in quite an important meeting at work, when I started to feel a strange sensation in my chest. I could sense my heart beating very fast and I felt slightly dizzy.

Initially all I could feel was a vague sensation of discomfort around my heart, which I did my best to shrug off, but it quickly progressed to a peculiar fluttering, almost as if I had a butterfly in my chest! That got my attention, and as I focused on the weird sensations, I was abruptly aware of my actual heartbeat, which seemed frighteningly fast. I became very anxious and left the office to visit my doctor immediately. The doctor said that I had experienced an episode of palpitations—probably brought on by all the coffee I had drunk over the course of the morning.

Just to be on the safe side, the doctor arranged for me to have an electrocardiogram at the hospital, to check that the electrical activity in my heart was normal.

Difficulties may arise when the tachyarrhythmia is intermittent, so that when the person undergoes an ECG, the heart is in a normal rhythm. There are various solutions to this problem.

- A 24-hour ECG recording can be obtained using a machine about the size of a personal stereo, which is worn on the belt, allowing complete freedom. If the arrhythmias occur even less frequently, longer recordings of up to 1 week can be made.
- For very occasional symptoms, the person may be issued with a device, again about the size of a small radio, which is placed on the chest, to take an ECG recording when symptoms occur. The recording can then be transmitted over the telephone line to the hospital for immediate analysis.
- For particularly infrequent but severe symptoms, such as blackouts every few months, for which no tachyarrhythmia has been documented, a further approach is electrophysiological studies. Electrodes are inserted into the heart via an artery and/or vein. The heart is then stimulated to cause the tachyarrhythmia, and the abnormal area of muscle is identified.
- An electrical device similar to a pacemaker can be implanted under the skin and is able to record the ECG for up to 18 months.

What are the treatment options?

There are two considerations in the treatment of abnormal tachyarrhythmias—to put the heart back into a normal rhythm and to keep it there. Restoring a normal rhythm can be achieved either by drugs or through the application of an electric shock, a treatment called cardioversion. In tachycardias that do not cause severe symptoms, drug therapy can be used to put the heart back into a normal rhythm and to prevent further recurrence.

In arrhythmias that are life-threatening or that do not respond to treatment, cardioversion is sometimes carried out. Under general anesthetic, a shock is applied to the heart via two hand-held electrodes placed on the front of the chest. Some supraventricular tachycardias are associated with an increased risk of stroke, so a blood-thinning agent (p. 115) such as warfarin may be prescribed for a few weeks before the rhythm correction is attempted.

Patients who experience episodes of ventricular tachycardia or fibrillation have recently benefited from the implantation of a specialized type of pacemaker called a defibrillator (p. 121). This device automatically delivers an electric shock to the heart in the event of an arrhythmia.

VARICOSE VEINS

A very common disorder, in which abnormally dilated and tortuous veins in the legs cause pain, and distress because of their appearance.

The veins in the legs form two groups—the superficial veins and the deep veins. The superficial veins lie just below the skin, whereas the deep veins lie within the muscles. The two groups are linked at several points by connecting veins. All these veins have valves, which ensure that blood flows in the correct direction, namely, from superficial to deep veins and then back toward the heart. Varicose veins result when the superficial veins of the leg become dilated and tortuous, so that they are visible on the surface of the skin as purple lumpy cords. The condition is quite common; between 10 and 20 percent of the population is affected—women moreso than men.

What are the causes?

It is widely believed that varicose veins develop because of poorly functioning valves within the veins. As a result, the blood flows in the wrong direction, from the deep to superficial veins. The increased pressure within the superficial veins then causes them to dilate. This is unlikely to be the whole story, however, and there is probably an inherent weakness in the walls of the veins themselves that predisposes them to distend.

Varicose veins often run in families. Pregnancy is a risk factor because the pressure of the fetus on the deep veins in the pelvis causes a backlog of blood in the leg veins. Varicose veins can also occur following a deep vein thrombosis that damages the valves.

What are the symptoms?

For many people, the main problem caused by varicose veins is cosmetic—The often large and visible veins can be unsightly on the leg. Other symptoms include the following:

- Aching pain in the affected region that is troublesome and can limit activities
- Eczema, which is intensely itchy
- Swelling of the leg
- Brown discoloration of the surrounding skin

More severe varicose veins can lead to the formation of small ulcers following a minor injury to the affected leg; these can be very painful and difficult to heal. Occasionally, clots form in one of the varicose veins, giving rise to a condition known as thrombophlebitis, characterized by pain, fever, and hardening of the affected vein.

Does a lot of standing cause varicose veins?

It has long been thought that people whose jobs involve a lot of standing—such as soldiers who stand at attention for long periods of time, hairdressers, or shop assistants—are more prone to developing varicose veins because of pooling of the blood in the lower legs. However, long-term standing probably only aggravates an existing problem. In other words, the varicose veins would have developed for other reasons, whatever the person's profession or standing habits.

ASK THE EXPERT

How is it diagnosed?

Diagnosis of varicose veins is quite straightforward by visual and physical examination of the leg. No special investigations are required.

What are the treatment options?

People with small, mildly problematic varicose veins may benefit from wearing simple compression stockings. For more troublesome veins, especially those that cause pain, skin discoloration, or recurrent thrombophlebitis, or those that are particularly unsightly, referral to a surgeon to discuss more serious treatment options is usually recommended.

Three main surgical therapies are available. The varicose veins can be injected with a "sclerosing agent"—a substance that causes the vein to shrivel and close off. This procedure can be performed without admission to hospital. Following injection, the leg is wrapped in a bandage for about three weeks to ensure that the vein stays closed.

The second technique involves tying off the superficial veins so that blood can no longer flow into them (p. 130). The third technique is surgical removal of the offending veins (p. 129). Small incisions are made in the skin at the top and bottom of the vein, then, using a specially designed tool, the vein is stripped from the leg. Admission to the hospital is required, as is a general anesthetic, and the legs may be quite painful for some time after the operation.

Index

Acknowledgments

Carroll & Brown Limited would also like to thank:

Editorial assistant
Charlotte Beech

Picture researchers
Richard Soar, Sandra Schneider

Production manager
Karol Davies

Production controller
Nigel Reed

Computer management
Elisa Merino, Paul Stradling

Indexer
Kathy Croom

3-D anatomy
Mirashade/Matt Gould

Illustrators
Andy Baker, Peter Cox, Susan Doyle, Jacey, Debbie Maizels, Gillian Martin, Mikki Rain, Philip Wilson

Photographers
Jules Selmes, David Murray

Thanks to the Clinical Effectiveness Group (Department of General Practice and Primary Care) at St Bartholomew's & Royal London Hospital Medical and Dental School, Queen Mary and Westfield College, London, for their permission to use the chart on page 41.

QuitNet can be contacted at http://www.quitnet.org

Photographic sources
1 John Bavosi/SPL
6 (*left*) Quest/SPL
(*right*) Alfred Pasieka/SPL
7 SPL
8 (*top left*) Michael Davidson/SPL
10 (*bottom left*) Dr Kari Lounatmaa/SPL
11 (*top right*) SPL
(*right*) Alfred Pasieka/SPL
13 Victor Habbick Visions/SPL
14 (*left*) Quest/SPL
16 (*bottom right*) BSIP PIR/SPL
18/19 Chris Bjornberg/SPL
20 (*top*) Prof P Motta/Dept of Anatomy/University, 'La Sapienza', Rome/SPL
20 (*bottom*) Images Colour Library
24 Telegraph Colour Library
30 Quest/SPL
30/31 Biophoto Associates
31 BSIP PIR/SPL
32/33 Manfred Kage/SPL
37 (*top, second from top*) GettyOne Stone
37 (*bottom*) The Stock Market
38 (*left*) Keith Saunders/Arena Images
40 (*left*) Telegraph Colour Library
42 Michael Davidson/SPL
44 BSIP Laurent/Cathy/SPL
46 The Stock Market
47 (*top*) Telegraph Colour Library
(*bottom*) Keith Saunders/Arena Images
48 Telegraph Colour Library
50 (*bottom left*) GettyOne Stone
(*top right*) Telegraph Colour Library
51 (*left*) Nick Veasey/Untitled
(*right, second from top*) GettyOne Stone
52 David Parker/SPL
54 GettyOne Stone
55 GettyOne Stone
56 (*top*) Nick Veasey/Untitled
60 Image Bank
61 Alfred Pasieka/SPL
65 (*right, bottom*) Telegraph Colour Library
73 Telegraph Colour Library
77 Telegraph Colour Library
78 Telegraph Colour Library
79 (*right, second from top*) Telegraph Colour Library
80 (*center*) Gary R. Bonner
(*right*) GettyOne Stone
82 (*top left*) Telegraph Colour Library
83 (*top*) Image Bank
(*second from top*) Telegraph Colour Library
(*second from bottom, bottom*) GettyOne Stone
85 (*top*) The Stock Market
(*bottom*) GettyOne Stone
88 Telegraph Colour Library
91 GettyOne Stone
92 (*left*) Ribotsky DPM., Custom Medical Stock Photo/SPL
(*center*) Department of Clinical Radiology, Salisbury District Hospital/SPL
(*right*) SPL
93 CNRI/SPL
96 Wellcome Trust Medical Photographic Library
99 (*left*) Gail Jones
100 Alfred Pasieka/SPL
103 MIG/medipics
104 Geoff Tompkinson/SPL
105 (*top*) Mehau Kulyk/SPL
(*bottom*) SPL
106 CC Studio/SPL
107 Volker Steger, Peter Arnold Inc/SPL
108 Oullette & Theroux, Publiphoto Diffusion/SPL
109 Ribotsky DPM, Custom Medical Stock Photo/SPL
110/11 Images Colour Library
111 SPL
112 SPL
115 (*left*) CNRI/SPL
(*right*) SPL
116 (*center*) CNRI/SPL
117 (*top*) BSIP Laurent/SPL
(*bottom*) John Bavosi/SPL
118 Carroll & Brown
119 (*top*) Will & Dent McIntyre/SPL
(*bottom*) BSIP Edwige/SPL
120 Lunagrafix/SPL
121 Department of Clinical Radiology, Salisbury District Hospital/SPL
122/23 Deep Light Productions/SPL
123 Michael Donne/SPL
124/25 Michael Donne/SPL
125 (*top left, right*) Michael Donne/SPL
(*bottom left*) Wellcome Trust Medical Photographic Library
(*bottom center, right*) Michael Donne/SPL
126 SPL
127 (*top*) M11/medipics
(*bottom*) Dan McCoy/Rainbow/medipics
128 Corbis
129 Wellcome Trust Medical Photographic Library
132 Telegraph Colour Library

Back cover (*center*) GettyOne Stone
(*right*) Dept of Clinical Radiology, Salisbury District Hospital/SPL